Healthy Kids

Also by Marilu Henner

Healthy Holidays

Healthy Life Kitchen

I Refuse to Raise a Brat

The 30-Day Total Health Makeover

Marilu Henner's Total Health Makeover

By All Means Keep on Moving

Marilu Henner

with Lorin Henner

Healthy Kids

Help Them Eat Smart and Stay Active—for Life!

Foreword by Peter S. Waldstein, M.D.,
Clinical Assistant Professor of Pediatrics, UCLA

ReganBooks
An Imprint of HarperCollinsPublishers

Grateful acknowledgment is made to reprint "113 Ways Sugar Can Ruin Your Health"
from *Lick the Sugar Habit* by Nancy Appleton.

A hardcover edition of this book was published in 2001 by ReganBooks,
an imprint of HarperCollins Publishers.

First paperback edition published 2003.

Designed by Kate Nichols

Illustrations by Lynnette Lesko Henner

The Library of Congress has cataloged the hardcover edition as follows:
Henner, Marilu.
    Healthy kids: help them eat smart and stay active—for life!
Marilu Henner.
        p. cm.
    ISBN 0-06-621112-3 (alk. paper)
    1. Children—Health and hygiene. 2. Children—Nutrition.
3. Teenagers—Nutrition. 4. Obesity in children—Prevention.
5. Physical fitness for children. I. Title.
RA777.H465 2001
613'.0432—dc21
                                                    2001031839
ISBN 0-06-052852-4 (pbk.)

03 04 05 06 07 RRD 10 9 8 7 6 5 4 3 2 1

To children everywhere

and their right to be healthy

Contents

Contents

Contents

Foreword

Starting a healthy lifestyle is not something you begin only after there is a problem. Proper diet and nutrition in early childhood are essential. A child's diet in the womb, during infancy, and as a toddler can have lifelong effects on his or her health. Researchers are showing that a baby's food preference can be traced to the womb. For the first six months of a baby's life, nutritional needs should be summed up in two words: breast milk. Human breast milk is perfectly designed for the building of infant brain tissue. It has six times the essential fatty acids of cow's milk. This is imperative since the type of fat a baby consumes at this stage can affect brain development and function. Babies are usually ready for solid foods after six months, but they should continue breast-feeding for at least a year. Unfortunately, only 15 percent of American infants reach that goal, and only six out of ten breast-feed at all. Mothers should also be concerned about what they are eating during this period. Infants can develop allergies to foods passed on through breast milk.

Children's food options get more interesting after their first year. Parents need to set good examples to guide toddlers through this new world they're discovering. Kids feel the allure of junk food almost as soon as they can stand up, and are more likely to follow good examples. So as parents, if we eat healthy, we shall teach the joy of good eating by setting a good example. I always end my checkups by explaining to the children that they are what they eat. Introduce your child to a wider variety of tastes. Parents must base meals on foods rich in nutrients, not just fat. It's not uncommon for me to get a cholesterol reading of 250 for a five-year-old!

I have seen a crisis develop in this country during my twenty-four years of private pediatric practice—childhood obesity. The percentage of obese children has nearly doubled in the last two decades. Obesity now threatens approximately one in three kids with long-term health problems such as diabetes, heart disease, hypertension, and some forms of cancer. It may soon rival smoking as the number one cause of preventable death.

Children's impulses have not changed in recent decades—social forces have. There has been a demise of home cooking concurrent with a sharp rise in fast food and video technology. The average child usually prefers video games over outside physical sports. The school system has drastically cut back on physical education programs, and the consequences have already cost us $100 billion in medial expenses and lost productivity.

Obese children suffer physically and emotionally throughout childhood, and statistics show that 75 percent will stay obese into adulthood. Genetics play a role in this, too. A lifestyle full of junk food and television often triggers obesity in children who are already prone to the condition. I see people every day in my practice who are in denial. They'll say, "My kid's not obese; he's eating healthy." When I ask what their child eats, they'll say, "Oh, we often go to McDonald's or we get a pizza for dinner." The days of Mom's home-cooked meals are over.

The problem, however, is not confined to home life. Some school cafeterias offer healthy foods, but because of short lunch periods and long lines, children often opt to dine on packaged food from the vending machines. Lunch is often nothing more than a candy bar and a Coke. Sugar is a leading cause of what could become an epidemic of childhood diabetes. There are two types of diabetes, Type 1 and Type 2. Type 2 is adult-onset diabetes, something that we formerly saw mostly in adults over forty. But now we're seeing it in young kids because their system, and particularly their pancreas, can't handle the amount of sugar that's being poured in daily. This sharp increase in adult-onset diabetes in children will eventually cause high blood pressure, kidney problems, or even kidney failure. Tragically, kids with diabetes don't generally heal well. Relatively simple infections can become very serious, sometimes resulting in limb amputations. It can be that heartbreaking.

Cow's milk and other dairy products are also a big problem. I frequently see patients with chronic ear infections and runny noses. The culprit is almost always dairy products. I usually advise parents to take their child off cow's milk. Invariably they return a month later with what appears to be a different child—no ear infection, no congestion, and no runny nose.

The time to get serious about childhood obesity is now, not in fifteen or twenty years, when today's kids are hobbled by coronary artery disease and diabetes. Families need to know when and how to intercede because there is always the danger that a child's obesity will be further complicated by anxiety, depression, or a life-threatening disorder.

Everything in life has a price. If these kids eat an unhealthy diet now, they will tragically suffer the consequences later. The two biggest risks of obesity are diabetes and cardiovascular disease. When I'm treating young children with high cholesterol, I explain to them how fat can get in the lining of their blood vessels and over time will make the openings in these blood vessels get smaller and smaller. After many years of fat accumulation, there will not be enough space for blood and oxygen to get to the tissue of the heart. The tissue will die, and that's how people get heart attacks. This can be difficult for a child to accept, but it's an extremely important lesson for a child to understand.

Learning to eat properly is as important as learning to read. This goes for parents, as well. Parents should learn as much as possible about diet, nutrition, and exercise, and set a good example for their children by eating healthy foods and exercising regularly. This book should be a great help to parents and children in their quest for a healthier lifestyle.

Peter S. Waldstein, M.D., F.A.A.P.
Clinical Assistant Professor of Pediatrics, UCLA
Attending Physician, Cedars Sinai Medical Center
Los Angeles, California

Acknowledgments

If it takes a village to raise a child, it takes a world of support to write a children's health book. With love and thanks . . .

To the incomparable Judith Regan, who is relentless in her pursuit of quality. Her unbeatable team at ReganBooks and HarperCollins—Douglas Corcoran (with thanks and appreciation), Renee Iwaszkiewiez, Cassie Jones, Renato Stanisic, Carl Raymond, Kurt Andrews, Lucy Albanese, and the brilliant Paul Olsewski, who makes every book tour better than the one before.

To Mel Berger, Rick Bradley, Sam Haskell, Jonathan Howard, and Gayle Nachlis of the William Morris Agency, Marc Schwartz, Rob Ree, and the fantastic team at Fusion Management, Dick Guttman and Susan Madore of Guttman and Associates, and Richard Feldstein and Barbara Barbour at Provident Financial Management.

To the talented and lovely Deborah Wald and her assistants, Arturo Everitt and Mark Leibowitz, for another wonderful photographic experience. And to Leslie Veje, Sarah May Wald, Ashley Lewis, Justin Sawai, Jacquelyn Feldman, Natasha Feldman, and, of course, the indescribable Sharon Feldstein who always makes us look good.

To all of the people of Marilu.com, who are helping to spread the THM word to families around the world: Mary Beth Borkowski, Sleeker, Tracey Beaver, Wendy K, Julie Bensinger, Robin Papa, Jenna Taylor, Audrey Winkels, Rosemary M.

Acknowledgments

Guidry, Geri, Erin Moore, Renee, Deborah McCloskey, Susan, Sheri, Valerie Durbin, Natashia M. Hope, Stephanie Hayes, Kathy Fena, Andrea Yolar, Edna Axelrod, Jan Van Ess, Lynn Kiel, Suzanne Palumbo, Allison Merriman, the One World Live team, and especially the fabulous Tonia Raebiger, who keeps it all together with grace, style, and composure. Thank you all for your Gusto!

To Adrienne Parsons, Paul Horowitz, and Nancy Whitson of the Buckley School. To Tracey Beaver, Steve Beaver, Robert Stem Jr.; and the Thomas B. Conley Elementary School in Asbury, New Jersey; Cynthia Giarelli, the faculty, and the seventh- and eighth-grade classes of St. Mary's, Lake Forest, Iillinois; Donna Viola and her valuable contribution, Gina Carney, and Beverly Carney. Thank you for all of the information you provided.

To Senator Paul Pinsky for his remarkable bill on vending machines and fast food in our schools.

To Ted Pastrick, MPT, for his firsthand knowledge of the physical well-being of children today. And to Susan Cole, PE teacher extraordinaire, for her time and expertise.

To Peter Waldstein, M.D., F.A.A.P., for his medical acumen, and to his wife, Laurie Waldstein, renowned author of several wonderful books, and to Dr. Mark Goldenberg, D.D.S. Thank you for your support and for keeping my boys healthy.

To Dr. John Seed and Rafael Sharon for their knowledge and support throughout the years.

To Dr. Ruth Velikovsky Sharon, the incomparable psychoanalyst, with gratitude for her insights and brilliance throughout the years.

To the best book team ever: Celina Carvajal, team rookie, for her personality, enthusiasm, and Web-surfing abilities. Working with you was a total joy (just ask my boys). To Brent Strickland for his energy, "can do" spirit, and valuable information as dad to his darling little girl, Madison. To the lovely Inara George, factoid queen, whose gentle elegance never failed to calm the storm and make us all smile. To Bryony Atkinson, whose razor-sharp wit and fast fingers kept us all together and on time. To MaryAnn Hennings for her incredible recipes and friendship. She does it all, looks like a babe, and is a working mom of two beautiful girls, Taylor and Madison. To Caroline Aaron and James Forman (writer extraordinaire), who were there to provide a wealth of information because of their fabulous children, Ben and Sydney. To Lynnette Lesko Henner, my gorgeous sister-in-law, whose creative abilities are as special as her musical talents. To Steve Lesko, her father, for his unending support. To Elizabeth Carney, my beautiful and talented niece, for her organization and ability to do anything and everything (and the best skin ever)! To the world's greatest coauthor, my brother, Lorin Henner, our sixth book together, and it just gets better. Thank you for everything you do, and for being so funny while you do it. I'm lucky to have you.

To Elena Lewis, for taking good care of everything around us. To Lissi Holmstrom for her wonderful help. To Donna Erickson, for her gentle, kind, loving nature, and the best edamame cook ever. To my stepchildren, Erin Othick and Lorne Lieberman, for being a wonderful introduction to motherhood. To my talented husband, Robert Lieberman, for being a great partner in parenting. And to Nicky and Joey, for being the best kids (and guinea pigs) I could ever hope for.

Introduction

There is nothing worse than a sick child. It is terribly frightening when your child is suddenly stricken with an unknown illness and you don't immediately know what to do to relieve their pain. I had a real scare in Seattle last year when my son Nicky, who was six at the time, had an allergic reaction to shellfish. At first he broke out with a mild case of hives. But later, after his stomach became hard and distended and he started crying and writhing in pain, I had him in a Seattle hospital emergency room within minutes.

The doctors put him through a series of tests, and after a few hours, they concluded that he was indeed having a severe allergic reaction to some shellfish he had eaten that afternoon at Pike Place Market. This was not the first time that Nicky had eaten shellfish, but it was the first time he had an allergic reaction. The doctors explained that a person could eat something twenty times and get their first bad reaction the twenty-first time. They hooked him up to an IV, and soon Nicky, completely exhausted but feeling better, fell asleep at around 2:00 A.M. When he woke up the next morning in that strange hospital bed and realized I had spent the night in the chair next to him, he very sweetly looked in my eyes and said, "Thank you, Mommy, for taking care of me." I can't help but cry every time I think about that moment. It was so special. It is moments like this when we parents realize that our children so completely entrust their health in our hands. It is our responsibility to make every effort we can to protect them and wholeheartedly stack the odds against illness in their favor.

If you are a parent, you already know that nothing matters more in this world than your children. We want them to be happy and healthy and smart and balanced and full of life! We want to keep their little immune systems as strong as possible to fight cold and flu viruses and all the other bad guys and diseases that cross their paths. And we want them to be wise enough to make the right choices for themselves when we are not there as they grow up and become more independent. We simply want them to have it all!

As parents we owe it to our children to ensure their health in every way we can. Unfortunately, today we face an onslaught of obstacles coming from every direction: a powerful fast food industry, endless junk food advertising, ridiculously "supersized" portions, more than 3,000 chemicals and food additives, misleading labels on packaged foods, school lunch program budget deficits, and profit-driven meat, sugar, and dairy industries. Not to mention the sedentary temptation of television and computer games, rampant growth of childhood obesity, lack of sense of community in our neighborhoods, and a world that's moving too fast for us to share quality family time and healthy home-cooked meals.

I became passionate about writing this book because as a mother for the last seven years and a stepmother for the last fifteen, I was never able to find a book about children and nutrition in which all the information I wanted was in one place. There were plenty of books about pregnancy and breast-feeding and babies and toddlers, but nothing covering the whole spectrum: play dates, fast food, school lunches, junk food temper tantrums, sleepovers, allergies, behavioral disorders like attention deficit disorder or attention deficit hyperactive disorder (ADD/ADHD), and childhood diseases like diabetes. I couldn't find a book that addressed how to train a child's palate to taste the vast and subtle flavors of real food so that he will no longer crave candy and junk food. These are trying times for grown-ups and kids trying to be healthy. Childhood obesity is at an all-time high and the age for puberty is at an all-time low. We have to look at the total picture to understand the state of health of our children.

I believe in a very simple equation: healthy food equals healthy kids.

In his 1988 Report on Nutrition and Health, C. Everett Koop, the surgeon general of the United States at the time, said, "Your choice of diet can influence your long-term health prospects more than any other action you might take." And your choice of diet for your child can influence your child's long-term health prospects more than any other action you may take as a parent.

Food provides the building blocks for a strong and healthy body and the energy your child needs to learn, play, and grow. Food also provides immediate information to the body. Food can make your child feel happy, content, and re-energized; or tired, jumpy, and irritable. Every breakfast, lunch, snack, and dinner provides the nutrient base for each cell in your child's body. There's no question about it—the nourishment a child receives in the womb, during breast-feeding, as a toddler, adolescent, and teen profoundly affect his health and his lifetime habits.

Children need whole natural foods to maintain health. We need to provide our kids with a variety of the freshest whole organic foods so their bodies can be healthy and develop fully. Whole foods are unrefined grains, beans, nuts, seeds, fruits, and vegetables. Whole foods are as close to the way nature provides them as possible. Another way to define a whole food is "food that has only one ingredient—itself." Your child's body relies on the nutrients from these foods for proper growth as well as mental and physical vitality. A deficiency of even one important nutrient can cause imbalances that can lead to serious disease.

The typical junk foods that are specifically marketed for children can hasten diabetes, hypertension, and heart disease. We naturally associate breakfast cereal with children. If you read the ingredients on the boxes of most cereals, you will typically find things such as corn syrup, partially hydrogenated soybean oil, red and blue dyes, sugar, and so many other refined sweeteners. For the most part, American breakfast cereals are nothing but chemicals and sugar. Our kids' lunches and dinners are not much different. It should come as no surprise, then, that 40 percent of the children in our country are severely malnourished. Many are actually malnourished *and* obese. The United States has, for so many years, prided itself on being the country that is most able to properly feed and nourish its citizens, but, because so many of our foods are overprocessed and stripped of their nutrients, we are no longer such a "nurturing" nation. In fact, many Americans are as malnourished from eating junk food as citizens from developing countries who do not have enough to eat.

I recently read a great article by Dr. Lendon Smith. In it, he mentions an observation a colleague of his, Dr. Howe, made during a trip with his sons to the San Diego Zoo. He noticed a sign near the vending machines that said, "Foods in the machines are for humans only. Do not feed this food to the animals or they may get sick and die." The veterinarians at the zoo obviously know that these foods will endanger the health of a 400-pound ape. What do you think vending machine "food" does to us?

Even our standard government-recommended food pyramid tells us that the majority of our diet should consist of fruits, vegetables, and whole grains. Because of this, most parents are content when they see their children eating breads and other starchy foods and carbohydrates (muffins, oatmeal cookies, etc.). But only 2 percent of the flour consumed in this country is whole grain. On average, twenty-four ingredients are removed during refining. So, the essential grains and nutrients we assume our children are getting from their pastas, breads, and muffins have been depleted during processing and refining.

The focus of my first book, *Marilu Henner's Total Health Makeover*, is about finding the B.E.S.T. diet and exercise regimen for you and helping you begin and maintain that regimen. B.E.S.T. stands for Balance, Energy, Stamina, and Toxin free. The book outlined the ten steps I took to improve my health. Since writing *Total Health Makeover* (or THM as people like to call it), I have connected with thousands of people all over the world who have been helped by the same information that helped me. This book, like the *Total Health Makeover*, is committed to finding the B.E.S.T. diet for your children *and* for you.

During pregnancy, breast-feeding, and your child's first few years, you, the parent, are pretty much in control and your focus is basically the same. But in the second half of *Healthy Kids*, when your child becomes more independent, your task becomes a lot more challenging. At that point this book will focus on helping you teach and inspire your children so that they will make healthy choices for themselves.

I'm hoping this book will be for you a condensed reference book and road map to spark your interest and understanding and help guide you and your family toward better health. I don't have to tell you that there is nothing more important than our children. They are not only our greatest joy in life, they are also the future.

Healthy Kids

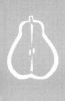

1

· · · · · · · · · · · ·

What's Happening with Children Today?

Does This Sound Familiar?

The alarm goes off, and you know you're about to face another day of battles. It's time to wake your kids up for school, but of course every time you go in there the kids want "five more minutes!" and then "just five more minutes!" You keep going into their rooms, but they are so groggy you finally have to drag them from their beds to the breakfast table. You give them Froot Loops or Lucky Charms or some other overly processed, super-sugared cereal. You finally get them up, but now they're so amped up, they're jumping around, out of control. You can't get them dressed. You finally get them into the car or to the school bus with a lot of screaming and fighting. At around ten o'clock they are crashing from their morning's first sugar fix, but not to worry. At ten-thirty, it's "Snack Time!" and the teacher or somebody has brought today's "healthy" snack, which is Fruit Roll-Ups or Capri Sun, or yogurts with sugar sprinkles or fruit cups with syrup or another white flour, white-sugared cereal. Now their midmorning fix is complete, and just as they're crashing again, it's time for lunch. But because they've already been on the sugar treadmill twice that day, do you think they want the fruit or the sandwich you've packed for their lunch? No way! They want a candy bar, or Coca-Cola, or anything else that is sugary to keep them on the treadmill, OR it's time for them to swing their pendulum in the other direction, to the salty side, so they crave pretzels, chips, or Goldfish instead. In no time at all, your kids are crashing after their lunch and can barely get through the afternoon's schoolwork. By the time you pick them up after school, they are ravenously hungry because they've barely had any food with any nutritional value at all. In fact, when you check their lunch boxes, the apples and sandwiches are still there, but there are candy wrappers letting you know they've eaten something.

But now they're in the car, and what do they want you to do? Stop at your nearest fast food restaurant, drive through as quickly as possible so they can get more salty food (French fries and a burger) and more sugar (Coca-Cola or Sprite). And just think, you can get it all in one little box with a toy thrown in for the kids to fight over during their *next* junk food crash.

Even if you don't drive through your local fast food chain, the first thing the kids do when they get home is hit the refrigerator and pantry for something equally "junk foody." It's their fourth fix of the day and by the time they're sliding down the other side of the sugar mountain, it's Supper Time! Of course they are barely going to touch their dinners because their palates, which have tasted only extreme salt or extreme sugar all day long, can't even recognize anything remotely healthy. There's so much fidgeting and complaining that you finally let them leave the table to go watch TV.

Within an hour, they want a snack while they're watching, which involves more salt (chips, popcorn, etc.) and more sugar (soda, cookies, ice cream, etc.). But anything to keep them quiet and calm, so of course you give in and let them watch TV while they mindlessly munch. You try to get them to do their homework, but they're too unfocused or too tired to concentrate, so you plan on having them wake up early tomorrow because guess what, it's time for bed—the biggest battle of them all! It starts with their saying that they're really, REALLY hungry, and because you know they haven't had much of a meal all day, you give them what they ask for, which is *another* bowl of cereal. So now, once again, for the sixth time that day, they're amped up. In fact, too amped up to go to bed, so it takes about an hour and a half after eight tuck-ins, seven "Settle downs!" six sips of water, five kisses, four "I love you toos", three bedtime stories, two trips to the bathroom, and one exhausted child who hasn't had a decent thing to eat all day. You finally get a few moments to yourself, but just before you close your eyes for some well-deserved sleep, you realize you get to do this all again tomorrow because your children will wake up with their white flour, white sugar hangovers.

In fact, if you think of the food your children have eaten that day, most of it is what is known as white food—white sugar, white flour, white dairy. There's very little color. There's hardly any green or yellow or orange unless it's green dye #3, yellow dye #5, or orange B (as in a hot dog).

We have to ask ourselves, "How did our children's nutrition get to this point?"

The State of Our Children's Health

To determine how and why our children's lives have developed into this scenario, we have to look at several factors that have jeopardized the health and well-being of our children in the past few decades:

- ✦ Exponential growth of fast foods, snack foods, and soft drinks
- ✦ Lack of exercise and a noticeable reduction in physical education programs in our schools
- ✦ Increased viewing of TV, video games, and computers
- ✦ Neighborhoods that lack sidewalks safe enough for walking or other forms of exercise
- ✦ A preference for riding in cars instead of walking or bicycling in even the safest neighborhoods

Big business, constantly striving to increase profits, has shaped our diets and the diets of our children, while our health and well-being have been all but ignored. Companies are giving us more sugar, more milk, more eggs, fatter chickens, fatter cows, faster food, more refined foods, more convenient meals, and foods that never spoil. And, because of this, our children and we adults are getting sicker, heavier, lazier, and emotionally crazier. Young girls are starting to menstruate years earlier than we did in our generation because of the dangerous amount of bovine growth hormones they are consuming secondhand from our meat and dairy supply. What are we doing to our children? Kids rarely eat fruits and vegetables or grains or beans or other whole foods. The consequences are that we are seeing unprecedented numbers of cases of asthma, juvenile diabetes, and cardiovascular disease in children, not to mention greater toxicity in our environment, which has in turn contributed to the increase in children's cancers and autism. Millions of kids nationwide are taking drugs like Ritalin to alleviate ADD and ADHD before even trying to change their diet, when we now have proof that diet and nutrition can do so much to balance a child's behavior. We cannot always move away from our environment if it is not healthy, but providing healthy food for our children is an area where we can exercise some control. Despite this, we are ignoring a simple equation:

Bad food = no energy = no exercise = laziness = depression = bad food

Here in the U.S. teenagers have too much of everything. And I don't just mean at private schools. Everything is at their fingertips. If they've got a car, they can get a video two minutes away and junk food is available on every block. Everything is too convenient and the portions are huge. These kids stuff themselves and don't exercise. You'll see them overeating junk food at sporting events or at parties. And you can't have any function in America without a lot of food being involved. To me, that's just such a waste of food and good health.—SUSAN COLE, PHYSICAL EDUCATION TEACHER

Here are some statistics regarding United States dietary habits:

+ For the first time in U.S. history, more people are classified as being "overweight" than "average." If this trend continues, our society will start to consider it average to BE overweight.
+ Obesity is up 50 percent since 1991.
+ 55 percent of the population is overweight or obese.
+ About one-fourth of American children are overweight, according to national statistics.
+ U.S. Department of Agriculture (USDA) statistics show that American total daily caloric intake has risen from 1,854 calories to 2,002 calories over the last twenty years. That significant increase—148 calories per day—theoretically works out to an extra fifteen pounds per year.
+ Today's average American diet is killing more than twice the number of people killed in World War I, World War II, the Korean War, and Vietnam combined, *EVERY YEAR!*

✦ U.S. Department of Agriculture believes that more than 80 percent of the American population eat too much saturated fat and too few fruits, vegetables, and fiber-rich grains.

✦ The average American eats over 200 pounds of sugar and artificial sweeteners per year (over 20 teaspoons per day).

✦ Carbonated beverages and French fries are the most commonly consumed food items outside the home.

✦ The U.S. population spends approximately $50 billion per year on weight loss, including low calorie foods and beverages. That's fifty times the money spent by the United Nations for hunger and famine relief.

✦ One in 3 Americans is on a diet.

✦ About 95 percent of the people gain back all their weight within the time it took to lose it.

✦ About $40 million a year is spent on advertising for over-the-counter diet pills.

✦ Surveys have shown that 1 out of 5 teenage girls between the ages of twelve and seventeen take over-the-counter diet pills and that 70 percent of young girls start dieting by the age of ten.

✦ Billions of dollars have been spent on research cures for diseases in this country; practically nothing has been spent on disease prevention.

✦ People are living longer because of medical advances; yet senior citizens take an average of eight prescription medications daily.

✦ Heart disease now accounts for 50 percent of all deaths, up from 40 percent in the 1970s.

✦ One out of 2 people eating the typical American diet eventually dies of cardiovascular disease, yet only 1 person in 25 dies of cardiovascular disease when eating no animal products.

✦ We are the first generation in history to experiment with thousands of potentially toxic chemicals in our food.

✦ Profit is the number one priority for every food processor in America.

✦ Food additives are rarely tested adequately because the government is understaffed, underfinanced, and controlled somewhat by powerful lobby groups. Because of this, dangerous carcinogenic additives continue to be used.

✦ A fetus cannot deal with foreign chemicals. Whatever toxic substances the mother eats flow largely unimpeded into the fetus. Unlike an adult, the fetus lacks protective, detoxifying substances. Teratogens are toxins that harm fetal development. Certain food additives are considered teratogenic.

✦ Each year in the United States an estimated 8,000 children are diagnosed with cancer. After injuries, cancer is the second most common cause of death in American children beyond the first year of life.

✦ We cannot predict what the long-term effects of food additives will be on today's children after a lifetime of exposure to chemicals that never existed before.

Obesity and Illness on the Rise

When I first talked about writing a book about children and health, people said, "What's the big deal? Aren't kids today better off than we were?" We now know the answer to that question is a resounding "No, they are not." You can't open up a *Time* magazine or *USA Today* or the health section in your daily newspaper without finding an article addressing the health of our children. Throughout this book, we will examine the various factors contributing to the health of our children. We look at each factor, starting with what Dr. Peter Waldstein, the pediatric consultant for this book, says is now a crisis—childhood obesity. And he's not alone. According to the U.S. surgeon general, David Satcher, "Childhood obesity is at epidemic levels in the United States. We have been remiss in shedding light on this problem, which leads to so many other health problems, particularly when we consider the threats this disease imposes on our children. Today, we see a nation of young people seriously at risk of starting out obese and dooming themselves to the difficult task of overcoming a tough illness." An estimated 300,000 Americans die every year because of obesity, and it is estimated that an additional 200,000 die of diseases that are related to it. That's half a million people. But what is considered "obese"? For adults, obesity is defined as being more than 30 percent over ideal body weight, but for a child it means greater than 25 percent—as little as ten pounds overweight.

Recent statistics show there are approximately 10 million obese children in the United States. The percentage of overweight children between the ages of six to seventeen years has doubled in the United States since 1968, with "overweight" being defined as 20 to 25 percent over ideal body weight. The most recent

National Health and Nutrition Examination Survey conducted by the National Center for Health Statistics from 1988 to 1994 found that 1 in 5 children in the United States is overweight. That's 20 percent!

Studies show that 70 percent of overweight kids ages ten to thirteen will be overweight and obese as adults. This is due to the fact that puberty is the worst time for a child to be overweight. If a child is overweight as an adolescent, he will face a lifetime of struggling with his weight. He can get it under control, but it will be much harder on him than if he gains weight at any other time in his life. Being overweight in childhood often causes psychological and emotional consequences because these kids struggle with self-esteem issues and are often victims of teasing from peers. This too often starts a difficult cycle of social isolation, emotional withdrawal, depression, inactivity, more overeating, and further weight gain. Comedians are cruelly dubbing today's kids "generation XXL." How could we as a nation have let something so important get so out of hand?

Several health problems are associated with obesity, and the dangers increase with the age of a child. According to *Exercise and Children's Health* by Thomas W. Roland, there are twenty-six childhood conditions associated with excessive body fat, including coronary artery disease, hypertension, arthritis, kidney disease, and especially childhood diabetes. The incidence of diabetes linked to obesity has increased significantly in U.S. children in the past few decades, according to the U.S. Department of Agriculture (October 1998). It is now a major health problem. Of particular concern is the fact that there is a sharp rise in the type of diabetes normally found only in adults. But now we're seeing it in young kids because their bodies and particularly their pancreas can't handle the amount of sugar that's being consumed daily. This sharp increase in adult-onset diabetes in children will eventually cause high blood pressure, kidney problems, or even kidney failure.

A study of 1,000 schoolchildren in Cincinnati showed an increasing incidence of Type 2, or adult-onset diabetes, the form of the disease that is closely linked to weight. In 1982, about 4 percent of children in the study had Type 2 diabetes. By 1994, the rate had risen to 16 percent. Most children developed it between the ages of ten and fourteen, researchers said, and the onset of the disease was directly linked to obesity. Other studies have found similar trends in other cities.

Overweight children tend to have readings in the highest levels of the normal ranges for their blood sugar, blood pressure, and blood fats. Each of these factors is used to indicate potential health problems. This was found in the Bogalusa (La.) Heart Study, an ongoing project funded by the National Heart, Lung and Blood

Institute. Researchers at Columbia University found that overweight children as young as three and four showed signs of elevated blood pressure and cholesterol. Dr. William Dietz of the Center for Disease Control and Prevention says, "There's a lag between the development of obesity and the chronic diseases associated with it. We're in that trough right now. Very soon we'll see the rate of cardiovascular disease among teenagers rising."

Overweight and obesity are known risk factors for

+ Diabetes
+ Heart disease
+ Stroke
+ Hypertension
+ Gallbladder disease
+ Osteoarthritis
+ Sleep apnea and other breathing problems
+ Some forms of cancer (uterine, breast, colorectal, kidney, and gall-bladder)

Obesity is associated with

+ High blood cholesterol
+ Complications of pregnancy
+ Menstrual irregularities
+ Hirsutism (presence of excess body and facial hair)
+ Stress incontinence (urine leakage caused by weak pelvic-floor muscles)
+ Psychological disorders (such as depression)
+ Increased surgical risk

> *Obese children (of both sexes) are at a greater risk to form coronary heart disease and arteriosclerosis, whether or not they lose weight as an adult.*
>
> **Harvard Growth Study**

Obesity has emerged as a major health problem worldwide during this century. Oddly enough, in the past fifteen years, the percentage of fat in the American diet dropped from higher than 40 percent to about 30 percent of total calories because of fat-free and low-fat foods, yet obesity in adults and kids has increased substantially during this time. Most of these fat-free products are highly processed and full of chemicals. Americans are eating less fat but somehow getting fatter. When a product is labeled fat-free, people are fooled into thinking that they can eat a lot of it and not gain weight. They can't. Most fat-free food is overly processed and has very little whole food or nutritional value. After consuming it a person is still hungry and not satisfied. Changes in food preparation are another reason why people are getting heavier. Before World War II, all food was prepared from scratch and was mostly consumed when in season. After 1954, when frozen food became popular, people were no longer restricted to seasonal choices. When the microwave oven was introduced in 1974, children started taking a more active role in choosing and preparing foods without Mom's help. It became possible for them to eat a dinner full of chemicals that had nothing to do with real food. And if they didn't "nuke" it for themselves at home, they could always hit their local fast food drive-through. Most experts agree that the fast food industry has been the number one cause of obesity in children in the last thirty years.

The number of kids who frequently eat outside their home is adding to this trend. And that number is growing every year. Thirty percent of family meals consumed in America are fixed outside the home according to national food surveys. Not only are these meals much higher in fat, sugar, chemicals, and sodium, the portions are much larger than at home, too.

Children are exercising much less. Less than 50 percent of American schoolchildren participate in daily physical education. Another big factor is the time kids spend watching television. Video games and computers also add to the problems of sedentary life. But watching television is not just a problem of kids being sedentary; it is also highly conducive to lots of snacking, and not healthy snacking. And we all know what that means—mindless eating without regard to whether their stomachs are full.

Thomas Robinson and his colleagues at Stanford University have studied the effect of reducing children's use of television, videotapes, and computer games. They discovered that they could cut a child's body mass index (BMI) by half a unit in children who watched between a quarter to a third less television and videotapes and played fewer computer games. The BMI measures weight in relation to a person or child's height. Learning your child's BMI will help you determine how serious your child's weight problem may be and offers a good start on a road to improved health.

A person's body mass index is the most common guideline used to determine whether he is underweight or overweight. An adult's BMI is calculated (weight ×
703)/height^2. But BMI is not calculated in the same way for children as it is for adults. As children grow, their body fat percentage changes over the years. The

interpretation of BMI depends on the child's age. Also, girls and boys have a different body fat percentage range as they mature. Therefore, BMI is age-specific and sex-specific.

Before you begin to calculate your child's BMI based on her weight and height, it's important that height and weight are measured accurately; otherwise the BMI won't be correct. I know your pediatrician does this, but kids change between office visits. To measure your child's height, make sure she is relaxed and standing straight, with her shoulders pressed against the wall and her heels pressed against the floor *and* the wall. Have her look straight ahead, as if she were looking directly into the eyes of someone exactly her height, while you take the measurement. Use a flat, stiff object, like this book, and lower it to your child's head while she is standing against the wall to mark her height. It's important that the book is lined up at an exactly 90-degree angle from the wall. Use a right triangle if you have one. Then simply measure the floor to the mark on the wall. When you weigh your child, do so after he's removed his shoes and heavy outer clothes. Below are what standard BMI charts are based on.

BODY MASS INDEX FOR AGES 2 THROUGH 20

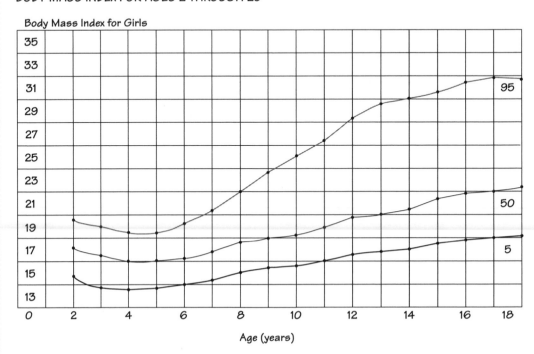

Body Mass Index for Girls

Body Mass Index for Boys

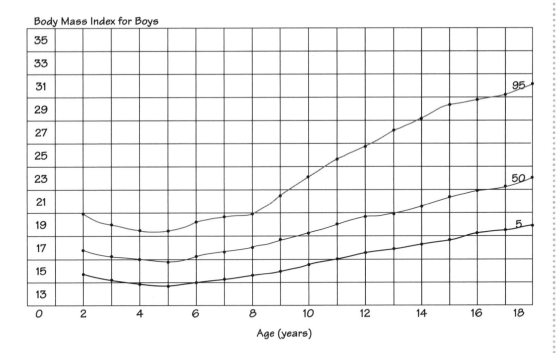

Age (years)

Use the tables as a rough estimate to determine if your child is overweight, and check with your physician.

The difference between a child's actual weight and ideal weight is divided by his ideal weight and then multiplied by 100 to get the percent that he is overweight. For example, an ideal weight of 120 with an actual weight of 150 would be calculated this way:

$$150 - 120 = 30$$
$$30 \div 120 \times 100 = 25 \text{ percent overweight}$$

General guidelines for children's weights are as follows (weights are in pounds):

+ birth (full term)—average weight = 7, lower limit = 5.5, upper limit = 8.5
+ 3 months—average weight = 13.2 male/11.5 female, lower limit = 10.2 male/9.7 female, upper limit = 15.5 male/14 female

- 6 months—average weight = 17.2 male/16 female, lower limit = 14.5 male/13.2 female, upper limit = 20 male/18.5 female
- 9 months—average weight = 20.2 male/18.7 female, lower limit = 17.7 male/19 female, upper limit = 23 male/21.5 female
- 12 months—average weight = 22.5 male/21 female, lower limit = 19.7 male/18 female, upper limit = 25.5 male/24 female
- 18 months—average weight = 25.2 male/24 female, lower limit = 22 male/21.5 female, upper limit = 29 male/27 female
- 2 years—average weight = 27.7 male/26.5 female, lower limit = 24 male/22.5 female, upper limit = 31.5 male/30 female
- 4 years—average weight = 37 male/35 female, lower limit = 31 male/30 female, upper limit = 43 male/41.7 female
- 6 years—average weight = 45 male/44 female, lower limit = 38 male/37 female, upper limit = 53 male/53 female
- 8 years—average weight = 55 male/55 female, lower limit = 48 male/45 female, upper limit = 68 male/70 female
- 10 years—average weight = 68 male/71 female, lower limit = 56 male/57 female, upper limit = 90 male/98 female
- 12 years—average weight = 88 male/92 female, lower limit = 70 male/72 female, upper limit = 112 male/123 female
- 14 years—average weight = 112 male/110 female, lower limit = 90 male/90 female, upper limit = 145 male/145 female
- 16 years—average weight = 136 male/123 female, lower limit = 112 male/100 female, upper limit = 172 male/158 female
- 18 years—average weight = 152 male/124 female, lower limit = 127 male/105 female, upper limit = 195 male/160 female

What's Happening at Home?

No Home-Cooked Meals from Scratch

When I was a child growing up on the northwest side of Chicago, it was a big deal to be the kid picked (out of six in my family) to go to one of the neighborhood stores. There were two, Freddy's, one block away, and Midwest, about three blocks away. You were allowed to go to Freddy's at age five (one street crossing) but had to wait until you were seven to go to Midwest (three street crossings). Safety was all about crossing the street and not about child abductions, like it is today. (The world was a safer place then; I think there were only three bogeymen in the entire country.)

Midwest had a much wider selection and was a little more glamorous than Freddy's which was only good for bread, penny candy, soda pop, and foot-long pretzels. If you could manage to scrounge up fifteen cents (usually from crevices in the couch or by returning empty bottles), you could get a Dreamsicle and a pretzel. If you could only find ten cents, you had to settle for a pretzel and a Push-up. The best part about Midwest was that our family had a charge account there that even we kids could use. All you had to say to owners Evelyn or Wally was "Charge it!" But you couldn't just walk in and charge candy and kid's stuff. That would be too obvious. My brother Lorin would get away with charging ice cream or barbecue potato chips because he would also charge up a grown-up item like Downey fabric softener to make it look good. Then he would simply throw the Downey in a trash can on the way home. What a waste! (Imagine all the kids in China with stiff clothes and no Downey fresh scent.) I have fond memories of those little neighborhood stores in Logan Square. You know, it's kind of sad. Today, every kid in America goes to the same neighborhood store, 7-Eleven.

Back then, there was also the big supermarket, National, that my mother would go to once a week on Thursday. She cooked from scratch for the most part, but would sometimes mix Campbell's soup with something like vegetables or ground beef. So, other than the Campbell's, we ate whole natural foods except for the one special, ultrachic, space-age food product we all looked forward to every Saturday night—Swanson's TV dinners! This was a big deal! Saturday night meant that we'd have a baby-sitter and a TV dinner. Every week, for the Thursday supermarket shop, we had to place our TV dinner order for that coming Saturday. I tried all the different choices. I think there were only four, but at the time it seemed like that's all the variety we'd ever need. My favorite was the turkey dinner because it had the cranberry sauce and stuffing. I also liked the fried chicken, and I remember having to fold back the aluminum foil for just the chicken section if I wanted it on the crispy side. I usually had to fold back the little dessert section, too, like the apple crisp. As wonderful as all this sounds, in reality, it was just the early stages of the junk food era we're in now. Working mothers spent less and less time in the kitchen cooking from scratch and began to enjoy the convenience of TV dinners. They were called as such because they were meant to be eaten in front of the television set. Nowadays the old TV dinners are just called dinner.

Hungry Man Dinners were the predecessor for supersizing. There is a big difference, however, between the ingredients in a typical TV dinner from the '60s and what our kids are eating now. As time went on, food manufacturers learned how to add more and more artificial ingredients to make their foods last longer and taste stronger. In those days, even fast foods like Arby's were made with real roast beef. You could actually watch the butcher (they didn't hire teenagers back then) slicing a huge, bright red rack of beef while you ordered. But fast food chains learned quickly how to increase shelf life and add exotic flavorings to increase profitability.

Most Food Is Processed and Convenient

The typical American family eats in a restaurant four or five times a week, despite the fact that each meal contains on the average 1,000 to 2,000 calories and fifty to one hundred grams of fat. Twenty-five years ago the average American family spent less than 25 percent of its food dollars on restaurant meals. Now, as much as 50 percent of those food dollars is spent going out to restaurants, and most of those are fast food restaurants. The average American today consumes approximately three hamburgers and four orders of French fries every week. The preparation of fast food shares very little with the traditional methods Mom or Grandma lovingly used to prepare foods at home. Practically all fast food is delivered to the restaurant frozen, canned, dehydrated, or freeze-dried. (It's like astronaut food, only worse!) Much of the taste and aroma of American fast food is now manufactured at a series of large chemical plants in New Jersey. (You know, the ones you can smell as you drive on the turnpike.) They've actually processed this "food" so much that they have to chemically put the flavor and aroma back in. For the most part, adults over thirty-five know that fast food can hardly be called food because they remember growing up during a time when mom-and-pop-owned neighborhood restaurants served real food and even fast foods were not as processed or full of chemicals as they are now. Unfortunately, our kids think that today's food is normal. Unless the typical American kid's current diet changes, her generation faces a lifetime of health problems associated with eating processed foods full of chemicals.

Whenever I think about chemicals in connection with food additives and added flavorings, I always remember the experiments we did during chemistry class in high school. Perhaps some of you remember this story from my second book, *Total Health Makeover*. Our teacher would give us beakers full of chemicals, and we would combine a few here with a few there. After mixing the liquids together, we were shocked when our teacher told us to take a taste of these concoctions. Most of my classmates refused, but my natural curiosity got the best of me, and because I liked and trusted my teacher, I volunteered to taste it. I couldn't believe it. Peppermint! Then we mixed a few more chemicals, and before I knew it I tasted strawberry and banana! How could this be? There was not a "real" fruit in sight, and yet here I tasted these very distinct flavors, and they were almost as real as eating the original. It dawned on me even then that this was probably the reason that so many children's medicines were these three flavors. Years later, when I was reading about chemicals in food, I remembered chemistry class and how we were able to synthesize flavors. It was a real lightbulb moment. Anything and everything could be made to taste like the "real" thing.

During the past twenty-two years, since I've been studying food and health, I've seen the amount of chemistry in our food go from bad to worse. Visit any grocery store and, at random, pick up a box of prepared food from the shelf and read the label. It's horrifying. I am always joking that you should not eat anything that needs a paragraph to describe it or says, "Continued on the next can." But when we are talking about giving this chemical-laden, sodium-heavy, sugar-sweetened, nutritionless food to our children—it's not funny. After doing the research for this book, I can honestly say without hesitation that the amount of chemistry in our food is killing us.

There is a wonderful best-selling book by Eric Schlosser called *Fast Food Nation* that uncovers the dark side of the fast food industry. Here is an eerie and alarming excerpt, in which Schlosser describes how fast food gets its "delicious" flavor:

About 90 percent of the money that Americans spend on food is used to buy processed food. But the canning, freezing and dehydrating techniques used to process food destroy most of its flavor. Since the end of World War II, a vast industry has arisen in the United States to make processed food palatable. . . . The flavor industry is highly secretive. Its leading companies will not divulge the precise formulas of flavor compounds or the identities of clients. . . . The New Jersey Turnpike runs through the heart of the flavor industry, an industrial corridor dotted with refineries and chemical plants. . . . The area produces about two-thirds of the flavor additives sold in the United States. . . . IFF's (International Flavors and Fragrances) snack and savory lab is responsible for the flavor of potato chips, corn chips, breads, crackers, breakfast cereals, and pet food. The confectionery lab devises the flavor for ice cream, cookies, candies, toothpastes, mouthwashes, and antacids. . . . In addition to being the world's largest flavor company, IFF manufactures the smell of six of the ten best-selling fine perfumes in the United States. . . . It also makes the smell of household products such as deodorant, dishwashing detergent, bath soap, shampoo, furniture polish, and floor wax. All of these aromas are made through the same basic process: the manipulation of volatile chemicals to create a particular smell. The basic science behind the scent of your shaving cream is the same as that governing the flavor of your TV dinner.—ERIC SCHLOSSER, *FAST FOOD NATION*

Doesn't this make you feel like we are living in a world with a big secret, like the movie *Soylent Green*?

Flavor and taste are not determined solely by the taste buds. We perceive taste through a complex process using our nose, taste buds, and brain (especially the brain stem and hippocampus). All three are necessary, and our sense of smell may be most important. It is rare when a person enjoys eating something she also feels has an unpleasant odor. Therefore, if food manufacturers can get the food smelling wonderful, then making it taste great should be a piece of cake—or should I say piece of ethyl vanillin and FD & C Red No. 40?

The Fast Food Conspiracy, aka "Pester Power"

The members of my family who have worked in the television commercial industry for years often talk about the "hard sell" and "soft sell" of advertising. Advertising agencies often use the term "pester power," which focuses on one of the primary objectives of child advertising—getting kids to nag their parents and to continue nagging them until they buy. Marketers even have categories for the different types of nagging kids do: pleading, persistent, forceful, demonstrative, sugarcoated, threatening, and pitiful. This is not just a marketing trick of the trade; it's developed into a science. And advertisers will continue to research children's behavior because attitudes and beliefs change from generation to generation.

The explosion in children's advertising began during the 1980s. Before that, only a few companies in the United States aimed their marketing at children. Children are recognized as a special audience and are considered easily influenced by each new mass media trend. And it's not just cereals, candies, and toys. Today, children are being targeted by clothing stores, phone companies, car companies, restaurant chains, and even oil companies. The music industry, in particular, has been targeting children for the last ten years. Researchers began noticing a trend in the 1980s among many working parents who felt guilty about spending less time with their kids. They compensated by spending more cash on them. Advertisers are well aware that children strongly influence their parents when it comes to product consumption, which is why child demographics get an enormous amount of corporate attention. Companies generally influence children with five popular techniques:

1. Selling the feelings of friendship and happiness. Products are always shown in a setting with friends having fun. It makes kids feel that they need this particular product in order to enjoy themselves, and if they don't have it, they unconsciously feel that everyone is having fun without them. This can make a child emotionally vulnerable. He may feel like a loser unless he gets this product.

2. Promoting product "popularity" is also a common technique. Advertisers will usually do a media blitz in order to create the illusion that their product is the most popular new thing that everyone must have. Popularity appeals to children.

3. Creating a series or a collection related to a product. Kids love the idea of collecting a series of something. Some kids become obsessed with collecting. Examples are Beanie Babies, Barbie dolls, and Precious Moments.

> **"P**arents should treat the media no differently than they would a stranger who knocks on their door and asks to come in to play with their children," advises Elizabeth Thoman, founder and president of the Center for Media Literacy in Los Angeles.
>
> *Parents,* November 2000

> **T**hirty billion dollars a year are spent on advertising and promotion for foods and beverages.
>
> *USA Today,* May 30, 2000

4. Getting endorsements from celebrities. Kids are enticed by products that are endorsed by popular athletes and celebrities. Kids want to be just like Michael Jordan or Britney Spears.

5. Using animated characters. In a survey done recently, 96 percent of American kids correctly identified Ronald McDonald. Only Santa Claus scored higher. A character on the McDonald's Web site talks about Ronald McDonald as being "the ultimate authority in everything."

The fast food industry is extremely powerful. More than 90 percent of kids between the ages of three and nine visit a McDonald's in a given month. (Sixty percent of McDonald's sales comes from Happy Meals, and twenty years ago they didn't even exist!) In fact, in polling thousands of children from five through eighteen, I discovered that over 40 percent of them visit a McDonald's or other fast food restaurant at least once a week. The main attraction here is not necessarily the food. Often it's the toys. The 1997 Teenie Beanie Baby giveaway was one of the most successful promotions in the history of American advertising.

The McDonald's Corporation was the single most heavily advertised brand (in any product category) in 1998, according to Competitive Media Reporting, New York. In second place was the Burger King Corporation. Taco Bell came in third place, followed by Wendy's and KFC. It's amazing that the top five spots were fast food companies.

How do parents compete with numbers like this?

Get Them While They Are Young

Market research has shown that a child's "brand loyalty" may begin as early as when she is two years old. In fact, children often recognize a brand logo before they can recognize their own name. What is really scary is that over 90 percent of kids over the age of six could identify Joe Camel in a 1991 survey, and it was found that one-third of all cigarettes sold illegally to children were Camels. Do you think that was just a coincidence? Or was it Phillip Morris's plan all along to "get them while they are young"? Remember: The tobacco industry "loses" more than 400,000 customers a year. They have to constantly find new users. As appalling as this is, how much better is fast food for our kids than cigarettes? Both are poison. Yet we don't think much about the fact that fast food chains advertise their products to children through toys, cartoons, movies, videos, amusement parks, charities, and playgrounds as well as through contests, sweepstakes, games, and clubs on television, radio, magazines, and the Internet. And now the fast food industry is actually advertising in the halls of our public schools. When advertising is all a child sees throughout her day, it simply becomes a normal part of her environment and the way she unconsciously defines food. There's no reason for her to think there's anything wrong with these products.

What's Happening at School?

School Lunches

School lunches today are not the same as they were even ten years ago. The biggest complaint of almost every kid I talked to was "no time." Most schools today allow kids only twenty to thirty minutes to scarf down their lunches, and because kids would rather use the time to socialize with their friends, the lunch they eat is whatever is fast and convenient rather than healthy and nutritionally dense. Because of this, vending machines are a serious problem in schools. Often kids will save a few dollars, and time, since there's usually no line for vending machines, by having just a Coke and a candy bar for lunch. That jolt of sugar gets them wired enough while they are hanging out with their friends, only to come crashing down when it is time to learn. And we wonder why our kids aren't learning the way we want them to. Over the last few years, while visiting school lunchrooms around the country, I was appalled at what most kids were eating. Often there was not one food that was real. They were primarily the same chemically enhanced, heavily sugared, overly salted, white-floured convenience foods that most kids eat all day long.

Two 1996 reports from the U.S. Department of Agriculture show that 13 percent of schools using the federally subsidized meal programs were serving brand-name fast foods and that students threw away about 42 percent of the cooked vegetables and 30 percent of the raw vegetables served to them at school. I am not surprised. Most of the vegetables that I have seen in school lunchrooms around the country are tasteless and/or overcooked. Current federal guidelines require schools to serve meals that contain no more than 30 percent of calories from fat and no more than 10 percent of calories from saturated fat, yet USDA surveys have found the average school lunch contains about 40 percent of calories from fat. I am always amazed that people are willing to pay premium for a gallon of gas, but complain that school lunch is expensive. The average price for a gallon of gas is $1.63. This gas will take your car an average of twenty-five miles, which is less than an hour of driving. The average price for a school lunch is also $1.63, but your child has to run on it the entire afternoon. As we have seen, the food our kids get for that $1.63 leaves them on empty in no time, yet the money invested in your car always gets you from point A to point B. Which do you think is a better investment?

Fast Food Takeover

The availability of fast foods on school campuses is skyrocketing. A recent California statewide study on fast foods in public high school found that 95 percent of the participating high school districts sell fast foods such as pizza, cookies, chips, and burritos, with Taco Bell, Subway, and Domino's Pizza ranking as the top three brands sold statewide. Entrées like pizza, chicken nuggets, and French fries are widely available at school. The American School Food Service Association estimates that about 30 percent of the public high schools in the United States offer brand-name fast food. Many elementary schools now serve food from McDonald's, Pizza Hut, and Subway. According to one school administrator, "We try to be more like the fast food places where these kids are hanging out. We want kids to think school lunch is a cool thing, the cafeteria a cool place, that we're 'with it,' that we're not institutional . . ."

Schools claim that the main reasons they allow fast foods to be served in their cafeterias are to financially support food service operations, improve school facilities, and support extracurricular programs. All in all, fast foods are cheaper and more profitable than more wholesome choices. Economics is the reason hospital food is so horrible, too. I always thought it was ridiculous that hospitals are built and operated to cure people and strengthen their health, yet they commonly serve junk food to their patients and staff because of budgetary restrictions. I'll never forget the time my aunt told me that the first meal served to her in the hospital after colon cancer surgery consisted of pork chops and chocolate cake. It's hard to trust a hospital that seems to disregard your basic nutritional needs.

At a recent press conference in California, Joseph Hafey, president and chief executive officer of PHI, a Berkeley-based nonprofit health organization that had commissioned a fast food study, said, "Fast foods on California campuses have become an epidemic. The irony is that in the same environment where we teach our students about health, we're encouraging them to eat their way to a future marred by heart disease, diabetes, cancer, and obesity. With teen obesity at an all-time high, our schools should not be fiscally forced to promote lucrative high-fat fast food over healthier options." Hafey called for school district officials and legislators to aggressively search for alternative ways of funding school and food service programs.

There was a bill recently proposed in the Senate titled the "Captive Audience/Stop Commercialism in Schools Act of 2001." This bill was intended to address "the increasing prevalence of product placements, advertising, corporate logos, and requirements for brand loyalty on school premises." It required "county school boards to adopt policies that clarify that students are not required to be exposed to commercial advertising outside of that which is necessary for instruction." Some of the other points included:

+ Prohibiting curriculum materials with brand names, logos, or other promotions unless that content is necessary for instruction
+ Ensuring that curriculum material is accurate, complete, and noncommercial
+ Prohibiting student access to vending machines until the end of the day
+ Prohibiting the requirement of students to participate in marketing surveys or provide personal information
+ Prohibiting county board policies that promote the use of particular brands of educational supplies
+ Prohibiting school uniforms with visible commercial logos or brand names
+ Requiring county school boards to adopt policies to discourage the consumption of candy, sweets, and other nonnutritional foods on school premises
+ Prohibiting agreements for the exclusive sale of vending machines and products on school premises
+ Prohibiting the posting of commercial advertisements on county-owned school buses

Unfortunately, according to Senator Paul G. Pinsky, "The bill was killed on second reading on the Senate floor by a vote of twenty-seven to seventeen with one excused."

Lack of Exercise

While the federal government asks schools to require daily physical education for all students, most states at the local level are not providing that, according to a report from the National Association of Sport and Physical Education and the U.S. Centers for Disease Control and Prevention. Less than 35 percent of children get daily physical education classes at school, and many no longer even get a daily recess. By ninth grade, 70 percent of girls and 50 percent of boys no longer participate in any type of vigorous physical activity at all.

Kids who get teased about their weight are going to avoid playing sports altogether and will often turn to activities that will not put them at risk for humiliation, like the Internet or television. That becomes their social life.

My sons' PE teacher, Susan Cole, feels that lack of exercise is perhaps a bigger problem than even bad nutrition.

I think inactivity is one of the greatest problems with kids today. Even if someone eats a lousy diet, they can still burn off some of the bad stuff by exercising. And the more you get involved with exercise, the more you begin to realize that soft drinks and junk food just don't do it for you anymore. You become more in tune with your body. Processed foods taste fake and you begin to crave things that are healthy and give you the most energy. I've noticed that kids who are active tend to be more conscious of how food affects them. I've heard even young kids say things like, "Oh, I shouldn't have eaten that greasy burger last night. My stomach's been upset ever since."

No Neighborhoods

In order for me to better understand our kids' current situation concerning physical education and recreation in our schools and communities in this country, I interviewed someone who works with children every day, renowned physical therapist Ted Pastrick. Here is what he had to say about the kids and neighborhoods today:

KIDS ARE NO LONGER IN CONTROL OF THEIR OWN PLAYTIME

Baseball legend Mickey Mantle felt that the creation of Little League in America was one of the worst things that ever happened to kids regarding the game of baseball because it created a structure to a children's game and took away neighborhood community and spontaneity. When he was growing up, kids would just get together of their own accord and would pick out a team, intuitively knowing who was good at which position. The kids themselves were in control of the game, not the parents, and they didn't have to wait for a 7:00 P.M. starting time. They were much more self-directed.

I believe this is the problem with the structure of the way kids play today. There is too much organization in a child's life. Kids now feel that activities have to be prearranged before they can do them. They have soccer practice, band practice, and scheduled play dates. They don't just simply play as we did in our generation. When I was a kid growing up in the sixties, playtime was like a nonstop decathlon with games like stickball, basketball, dodge ball, and running bases. Today, even if kids wanted to be more spontaneous with their playtime, they couldn't because other kids are in the same structured predicament. So they can't really break out of this. Kids no longer have the ability to spontaneously organize. Worst of all, kids are no longer in control of their own playtime. It's a systemic problem.

TV, Video Games, and the Internet

Time that used to be spent actively playing and exercising is now spent idly in front of a computer, video game, or TV. The Internet has added to the reduction of physical activity. And it's hard to get kids to stop because not only do they seem to be obsessed

The Henry J. Kaiser Family Foundation found that the more time children spend with the media (more than four hours a day for the average 8-year-old), the less content they are with their lives—as measured by how they perceive relationships with their parents and friends and how often they feel bored or sad, among other indicators.

Parents,
November 2000

Researchers at Baylor College of Medicine recently found that overweight children eat 50 percent of at-home dinners in front of the TV, while normal-weight kids do so only 35 percent of the time.

Parents, March 2001

with TVs and computers, but it also gives parents a break. So they unconsciously encourage it because it's a free baby-sitter.

On average, kids watch two to three hours of TV a day or twenty-one hours a week, not counting computer or video game time. In the course of a year, an average child watches more than 30,000 TV commercials. The federal government has taken an interest in the role TV plays in childhood obesity. Dr. David Satcher, the U.S. surgeon general, opened a speech recently at the National TV Turnoff Week by saying, "We have the most sedentary generation of young people in American history." National TV Turnoff Week is a campaign started by the nonprofit group TV-Free America. It's designed to get kids to stop watching TV and start moving and exercising. Dr. William Dietz, director of the Division of Nutrition and Physical Activity at the Center for Disease Control (CDC) in Atlanta, said, "Television-watching isn't simply a sedentary behavior, it also affects food intake." Fast foods are heavily advertised during children's TV programs, and advertising profoundly affects the amount and type of foods that children and teenagers choose. Thirty-five percent of an average family's meals are takeout food.

The Exercise/Calorie Chart for Kids gives some alternatives to watching television.

The Environment

The Effect of Pollution and Chemicals on a Child

An odd phenomenon has occurred over the last century. It's a bizarre sort of "good news/bad news" trend of major proportions in our history. The good news is that the infectious diseases that have plagued our planet for thousands of years have been significantly tamed during the twentieth century and are relatively under control today, thanks to the development and distribution of vaccines and antibiotics, better housing, safer drinking water, and improved sanitation. The ancient deadly diseases such as measles, smallpox, poliomyelitis, cholera, and many other

EXERCISE/CALORIE CHART FOR KIDS

Minutes	Activity	40 Lbs.	60 Lbs.	80 Lbs.	100 Lbs.
40	Taking gym class	58	89	122	151
30	Basketball	77	115	154	192
30	Ice skating	67	101	134	168
30	Riding a bike	67	101	134	168
45	Planting a garden	65	97	130	162
20	Hockey	51	77	102	128
30	Baseball	67	101	134	168
20	In-line skating	45	67	90	112
20	Sledding	45	67	90	112
30	Playing a game	38	58	77	96
20	Cowboys and Indians	29	43	58	72
20	Playing Barbie dolls	26	38	51	64
20	Dodgeball	77	115	154	192
20	Skateboarding	32	48	64	80
30	Making a snowman	29	43	58	72
20	Hide and seek	26	38	51	64
20	Skipping stones	26	38	51	20
20	Catching lightning bugs	26	38	51	64
15	Dancing around the house	26	38	51	64
20	Playing tag	29	43	58	72
10	Pillow fights	24	36	48	60

Minutes	Activity	40 Lbs.	60 Lbs.	80 Lbs.	100 Lbs.
	EXERCISE/CALORIE CHART FOR KIDS *(continued)*				
15	Running	38	58	77	96
15	Razor scooter	24	36	48	60
20	Taking a bath	22	34	45	56
20	Throwing snowballs	19	29	38	48
15	Bouncing a ball	19	29	38	48
15	Mother May I?	19	29	38	48
60	Playing Nintendo or PlayStation	16	24	32	40
20	Cooking and helping Mom with dinner	16	24	32	40
15	Jumping on the bed	16	24	32	40
20	Jump rope	16	24	32	40
20	Water balloon fight	22	34	45	56
20	Hopscotch	16	24	32	40
10	Chasing butterflies	13	19	26	32
10	Hula hoop	13	19	26	32
20	Duck duck goose	22	34	45	56
45	Doing a puzzle	11	16	22	27
5	Climbing a tree	16	24	32	40
5	Teasing your brother	8	12	16	20
15	Time-out	5	8	11	13
20	Eating	8	12	16	20
30	Watching TV	7	11	14	18

Minutes	Activity	40 Lbs.	60 Lbs.	80 Lbs.	100 Lbs.
	EXERCISE/CALORIE CHART FOR KIDS				
10	Walking the dog	7	11	14	18
1	Walking upstairs	7	11	14	18
10	Tickle fight	6	10	13	16
2	Taking the garbage out	6	10	13	16
5	Hunting for Christmas presents	16	24	32	40
1	Running for the bus	6	10	13	16
5	Helping Mom with the groceries	6	10	13	16
2	Brushing your teeth	6	10	13	16
5	Setting the table	6	10	13	16
2	Climbing on your mommy	6	10	13	16
30	Laughing	4	6	8	10
2	Changing as quickly as you can	3	5	6	8
3	Making your bed	2	3	4	6

diseases have finally been conquered or at least brought to their knees. The expected life span of an infant born today in the United States is more than twenty years longer than it was for a baby born at the beginning of the last century. That's the good news. Actually, I don't mean to downplay this. IT'S GREAT NEWS! But . . . that's not the whole story. There's another side to what has occurred in the last hundred years (especially the last fifty) that has profoundly affected the health of our children.

Children today face hazards that were neither known nor even imagined a few decades ago. There are 15,000 high-production-volume synthetic chemicals being used today that cause a potential exposure risk to everyone, especially to kids. Nearly all of these have been developed in just the past fifty years. Before that, they didn't even exist. More than half of these previously unknown substances are untested for toxicity.

The most serious diseases facing children today are chronic and disabling. There is even a specific term for this situation. It's called the "new pediatric morbidity." We have seen an increase in leukemia and brain cancer, twice as many deaths from asthma, widespread abnormal development of the nervous system, and the occurrence of hypostasis (poor or stagnant circulation in a dependent part of the body or organ) has doubled.

The exact cause of this new pediatric morbidity is not yet known. Childhood cancers and other environmentally related diseases are rapidly increasing, even doubling, and we're not even sure why. Well, I think I know why. We lack even basic information about the toxicity potential for most of the U.S. Environmental Protection Agency's list of approximately 3,000 industrial chemicals found in consumer products and the workplace. And the same goes for the 15,000 high-production-volume synthetic chemicals being produced in the United States each year for "other" uses. And, believe it or not, there are about 70,000 remaining chemicals on the EPA's inventory list. The EPA has initiatives under way to address the risks posed by some of these commercial chemicals, but this probably doesn't mean a whole lot since they have barely scratched the surface on testing the chemicals that are being used right now. It's possible that the EPA is really trying to do its best, but that this task is simply out of control. The reason we know so little about the role of environmental carcinogens in childhood cancer is because it's nearly impossible to pinpoint a culprit when there are thousands of variables. But I'm not saying we should give up trying. I believe we should support every effort the EPA is trying to make. The issues they seem to be focused on most right now are initiatives specifically addressing children's risks for cancer. At least that makes me feel a little better.

It is important to know that children are much more vulnerable to toxicity in the environment than adults. This conclusion is based on a detailed analysis done by the National Research Council in Washington, D.C., and is supported by the following factors:

Children have greater exposure to environmental toxicants than adults. Pound for pound of body weight, children drink more water, eat more food, and breathe more air than adults. For example, children in the first six months of life consume seven times as much water per pound as does the average American adult. Children one through five years of age eat three to four times more food per pound than the average adult. In addition, children have unique food preferences. For example, the average one-year-old drinks twenty-one times more apple juice and eleven times more grape juice and eats two to seven times more grapes, bananas, pears, carrots, and broccoli than the average adult. (Another good reason to buy organic produce!) The air intake of a resting infant is twice that of an adult per pound of body weight. Two behavioral characteristics of children further magnify their exposures to toxicants in the environment: their hand-to-mouth activity, which increases their ingestion of any toxicants in dust or soil, and their habit of playing close to the ground.

Children's metabolic pathways, especially in the first months after birth, are immature compared with those of adults. A child's ability to metabolize, detoxify, and excrete many toxicants is different from that of an adult. In some instances, children are actually better able than adults to deal with environmental toxicants. More commonly, however, they are less able to deal with toxic chemicals and thus are more vulnerable to them.

Children are growing and developing very rapidly, and their delicate developmental processes are easily disrupted. Many organ systems in young children—the nervous system in particular, but also the lungs, the immune system, and the reproductive organs—undergo extensive growth and development throughout pregnancy and in the first months and years of extrauterine life. During this period, structures are developed and vital connections established. These systems are not well adapted to repair any damage that may be caused by environmental toxicants. Thus, if cells in the developing brain, immune system, or reproductive organs are destroyed by *neurotoxicants,* or if *endocrine* disruptors divert development, there is high risk that the resulting dysfunction will be permanent and irreversible. Depending on the organ damaged, the consequences can include loss of intelligence, immune dysfunction, or reproductive impairment.

Because children have more future years of life than most adults, they have more time to develop chronic disease that may be triggered by early exposures. Many diseases that are triggered by poisons in the environment can take decades to develop. Examples of this include mesothelioma (cancer affecting the chest or abdominal cavity) caused by exposure to asbestos; leukemia, caused by benzene; breast cancer that may be caused by intrauterine exposure to DDT; and certain chronic neurological illnesses. These diseases are now thought to take many years to evolve from first exposure to development of the illness. Toxic exposures sustained early in life appear more likely to lead to disease than similar exposures received later in life.

There is very strong evidence that all of us have absorbed much toxicity from today's environment. In studies conducted by Caltech (California Institute of Technology), it was revealed that on average we have five times the amount of lead in our bodies than the amount found in prehistoric man. What's scary is that it has been estimated that it would take only four times our current concentration level to reach a toxic level. That is why there has been a strong movement toward getting lead out of substances like paint and gasoline. Heavy metals like lead can build up in our bodies. Luckily, there are certain foods that can aid in the removal of chemicals and heavy metals. Foods high in soluble fiber like beans, peas, apples, pears, oat bran, and corn seem to adhere to heavy metals and reduce their content in the body. These foods also have been found to lower cholesterol and help strengthen the body to fight cancer; so give them high priority on your grocery list for your family.

2

The Health Robbers

Sugar

The most common bad rap that sugar gets is that it gives you "empty" calories. You will often hear people say, "I don't think sugar is really that bad for you. It's just that it doesn't really do your body any good, so it's an empty food source. And if it helps my children eat the wholesome healthy foods they would normally avoid, what's the harm?" Believe me—sugar is far from innocent. In countless studies, it has been blamed for hyperactivity, diabetes, hypoglycemia, severe mood swings, decreased brain function, serious digestion problems, yeast infections, obesity, and tooth decay. It depletes your body of all the B vitamins. It leaches calcium from your hair, bones, blood, and teeth, interferes with the absorption of calcium, protein, and other important minerals in the body, and retards the growth of valuable intestinal bacteria. And that's not all! Sugar has a fermenting effect in your stomach. It stops the secretion of gastric juices and inhibits the mouth's ability to digest. Finishing even the healthiest of meals with a sugary dessert creates conditions in your child's stomach that are similar to those in a cheap winery.

> Today, the average American eats over 200 pounds of sugar and artificial sweeteners per year (over 20 teaspoons per day).
>
> www.parentsplace.com

Our bodies have several built-in systems that go into action when we introduce a heavy load of sugar into them. Minerals such as sodium, potassium, magnesium, and calcium from our bones are mobilized and neutral acids are produced in an effort to return the acid-alkaline balance of the blood to a more normal state. Consuming a fair amount of sugar each day continuously creates an overly acidic condition, so that more and more minerals are required from within our bodies to create this balance. Eventually, so much calcium is robbed from the body, bones, and teeth that decay and weakness result. As I have always maintained, it is not so much the calcium from dairy products that people need, but rather, they need to stop eating sugar to avoid the damage it causes to bones. Excessive amounts of sugar can eventually affect every organ in the body. At first, sugar is stored in our liver as glucose, which is the most common sugar and the main fuel for muscle contractions. The consumption of excessive refined sugar often makes the liver expand like a balloon since the liver's capacity is limited. Excess glycogen (the main form of glucose storage in the body) returns to the blood in the form of fatty acids when the liver gets filled to capacity. These fatty acids get stored throughout the body, especially in the most inactive parts: the stomach, butt, breasts, and thighs. (Now you know why you feel the way you do the day after a sugar binge!)

When these inactive "fatty" body parts get filled, fatty acids begin to find their way into our more vital organs, such as the heart and kidneys. This causes those organs to slow down, and their tissues eventually degenerate and turn to fat. The whole body is affected when the production of these organs slows and blood pressure often becomes abnormal. When you give up sugar, your body may have a withdrawal reaction at first, but after four days, you will not believe the sense of calm you and your children will feel. I have never seen it fail that people who stop eating sugar describe a sense of well-being as this "poison" leaves their system. In fact, when sugar is removed from the diet, even symptoms often associated with diabetes, cancer, and heart disease can disappear.

Brain function is also affected by an excessive consumption of sugar due to sugar's influence on the parasympathetic nervous system, which affects the small brain. What happens is that the circulatory and lymphatic systems can become invaded, and the balance and quality of the red corpuscles change. An overabundance of white cells is created, and our body's tissue-building mechanisms slow down. Our body's tolerance and immunity weakens, and we have difficulty handling extreme temperatures and viral and bacterial invasions. We can even have a difficult time handling insect bites. Pay attention to how much sugar your children eat and how often they get sick. There is definitely a connection.

> **M**ore than 15 billion gallons of soft drinks were sold in 2000.
>
> *Science News,*
> *February 28, 2001*

B vitamins play a key roll in brain function and digestion. Since sugar depletes the B vitamins, calculation, memory, and digestion are all affected by excessive sugar taken daily. That is why your child may have a difficult time concentrating after a sugar-loaded lunch. Keep a food diary for a few days. Write down everything your children eat. I bet you'll be surprised at how much sugar is in their diet.

A 1998 report from the Center for Science in the Public Interest identified soft drinks like Coke and 7Up, also known as "liquid candy," as the main culprit behind rapidly increasing sugar consumption rates worldwide that are "fueling soaring obesity rates" among youth. Soda consumption has doubled in the past two decades, making it the most popular kids' drink. The Center for Science in the Public Interest, a consumer interest group based in Washington, D.C., reported that the average teenage boy consumes three 12-ounce cans of soda daily, and the average teenage girl drinks about two cans daily. That's almost double what it was twenty years ago.

A study published in *The Lancet*, a British medical journal, in February 2001 found a significant and direct link between the number of soft drinks a child consumed every day and her likelihood of obesity. The study measured BMI (body mass index), which, as explained in Chapter 1, is a common measurement that is based on both weight and height. The study tracked over 500 eleven- and twelve-year-old kids from public schools in Massachusetts over two school years (1996 and 1997) and found that each sugared soft drink a child consumed daily at the beginning of the study contributed 0.18 points to her BMI. Later, if she increased her daily soft drink consumption, each extra soda increased her odds of becoming obese by 60 percent, regardless of how many sodas she was drinking before. Every child was already drinking at least some soft drinks at the beginning of the study,

> The sugar industry is big: $100 billion per year. As with any other billion-dollar business, there's bound to be a ton of information that will support such an empire anywhere you look—the media, bookstores, advertising, etc.
>
> Dr. Tim O'Shea,
> "Sugar, the Sweet Thief of Life"

> How many people do you know who drink at least one 12-ounce soft drink per day? If the sugar from each bottle could be crystallized, it would amount to 10 teaspoons.
>
> Dr. Tim O'Shea,
> "Sugar, the Sweet Thief of Life"

but the researchers concluded that the 60 percent per drink risk factor would remain constant, even if a child went from drinking none to one a day.

Soft drinks tracked in the study included regular sodas, Hawaiian Punch, lemonade, Kool-Aid, sweetened iced tea, and other sugared fruit drinks. It should be noted that pure 100 percent fruit juice was also tracked in the study and was found NOT to have the same obesity link as sugar-sweetened drinks. All in all, the study concluded that the odds of becoming obese increased significantly with each daily serving of sugar-sweetened drink.

Our country's three major beverage manufacturers (Coca-Cola, Pepsi, and Cadbury Schweppes) spend a great deal of money finding ways to boost sales of their soft drinks to American children. It has been very difficult for these companies to increase consumption among adults, so they turned their sights on our kids. Coca-Cola recently set a goal to increase sales nationwide by 25 percent a year. This is scary when you consider that kids are already drinking two to three cans a day.

White Flour

Refined white flour grains are really "empty" food. They are much less nutritious than whole grains. A grain is whole and unrefined if the entire kernel is left unaltered and intact. There are three parts to a whole grain: the endosperm, germ, and bran. The endosperm contains mostly starch and protein. The germ is rich in unsaturated fats, protein, carbohydrates, vitamin E, and B-complex vitamins and minerals. And the bran has a large density of fiber and contains minerals and B vitamins. During refining, the germ and bran are both removed, leaving only the endosperm. This process removes the most nutritional portion of the grain, including precious compounds and plant sterols that are helpful in disease prevention.

Today, nearly all grains are refined for greater marketability. The most common, refined white flour, is used in breads, bagels, rolls, sweet baked goods, most crackers, and cereals. Often manufacturers will add back some of the vitamins and minerals that have been removed, especially in some white breads and most children's cereals so they can make more impressive nutritional claims for their products. This does not make the grain whole again. Many other elements have been removed and lost through refinement. You cannot alter nature and expect to reassemble it to be what it was before. Adding vitamins and minerals only compounds the problem because it involves even *more* processing. Nature created whole grains with nutrients and protective compounds naturally built in that work together to provide all our bodies' needs. Enriched grain products rob your child's body of essential nutrition and confuse its natural processing and digestion.

There has been a lot of debate lately about the role carbohydrates play in our diet, health, and weight control. A few books have come out recently claiming that carbohydrates are bad for you because they raise your blood sugar: The theory behind this is that when your blood sugar rises, your pancreas creates insulin to bring your blood sugar back down. This increase of insulin accelerates the conversion of calories into fat, which in turn makes you fatter and over time adds to your risk of arteriosclerosis. Unfortunately, many of these books are saying that ALL carbohydrates do this and recommend a diet that consists primarily of high protein and high fat foods like (believe it or not) bacon, sausage, hamburgers without the bun, and even pork rinds as a snack. But many of these books fail to mention one of the most important points, which is that COMPLEX carbohydrates DO NOT provoke this insulin response! I had to uppercase those three words because it's so important to know that distinction.

Complex carbohydrates are whole grains, fruits, vegetables, and beans in their natural form. The fiber, grain, bran, and hull of these whole foods act to slow the body's absorption of food. So, instead of getting a quick rise in blood sugar and insulin and a storage of fat, you get a slow, steady rise in blood sugar, which gives you an even source of energy throughout the day. Simple carbohydrates (sugar, fructose, white flour, and even alcohol) cause a sharp rise in blood sugar, which leads to an insulin response, which leads to fat storage and weight gain.

The point is to feed your kids a diet that consists primarily of carbohydrates. Just make sure they are *complex* carbohydrates.

Wanting to eat products made with whole grains is one thing; determining which products are whole grains and which are refined is another. This is sometimes difficult. Some food companies will try to make you think you are buying something that

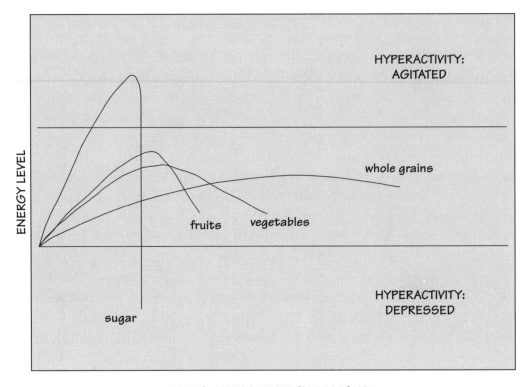

CARBOHYDRATE ENERGY RESPONSE

is whole grain when, in fact, it is refined. If a whole grain is listed first, the bread is mostly whole grain. Whole wheat, oats, amaranth, barley, buckwheat, millet, and popcorn are whole grains. Most flours are refined. If the label says "made with whole wheat," the product is often refined. If you find labels that list cracked wheat, multigrain, oat bran, seven- or nine-grain, stoned wheat, wheat, rye bread, wheatberry, or whole bran, you are looking at mostly refined grains. Try to eat sprouted grain bread as often as possible, and when baking at least use unbleached flour.

Most pastas in grocery stores, and even health food stores like Whole Foods, are not whole grain. However, there are many more whole grain pastas available than before. Read labels carefully and look for whole wheat pasta. There are also pastas made from buckwheat, amaranth, spelt, quinoa, and other grains that are excellent! Some cereals found in a typical grocery store that are made from whole grains. These include oatmeal, Shredded Wheat, and Wheatena. It may not always be possible for you to give your child whole grains and products made from whole grains, but you should try to avoid refined flour products as much as you can.

Meat

The typical American diet of children and teens (cheeseburgers, pizza, milkshakes, and fried chicken) begins clogging arteries as early as age two and will later contribute to heart disease, diabetes, strokes, and obesity. A study done by the department of medicine in Louisiana State University showed that yellow fatty streaks and cholesterol accumulations of significant amounts were found in most children under the age of five and in some infants as young as nine months old. The culprit: meat and dairy products consumed during pregnancy and early childhood. These streaks and accumulations are both strong factors for determining future arteriosclerotic clogging of the arteries. Eating grains and legumes instead of animal flesh and fats is great for both the mother and the child because helps the child develop a preference for foods that will promote a longer, healthier, more vibrant life. Add to this clean arteries, a much lower risk of cancer, and a much leaner and more attractive appearance. This kind of diet will obviously improve the health and appearance of the mother as well.

There is still a common belief that pregnant moms and growing children need to eat a lot of meat and dairy in order to get a large amount of protein and calcium. It is true that extra protein and calcium are important for pregnant moms and children; but, meat and dairy products are not the best sources of both protein and calcium. Plant foods (fruits, vegetables, legumes, and whole grains) alone contain more protein and calcium than a mom and baby will ever need. And you certainly don't have to eat meat to obtain a sufficient amount of protein. The female hormone estrogen and its synthetic, stilbestrol, are commonly found in beef and chicken. They are fed to the animals to increase weight, egg production, and fat content. They can be dangerously potent in the tiniest amounts, yet every time a pregnant woman eats a cheeseburger or milkshake, these hormones are being passed through the tissues of the developing brain and other vital organs of the fetus.

So many people believe that people must eat cow's meat or other animals for protein. But, think about this: what does a cow eat to produce that protein? Well, obviously the answer is grass! Cows should *never* eat

> Children eating the typical American diet today are going to be the heart patients of the year 2020.
>
> Charles Atwood, M.D.,
> *Dr. Atwood's Lowfat Prescription for Kids*

any animal meat. Protein is found in all green leafy vegetables and, in fact, in *all* living plants. It was once believed that in order for vegetarians to get complete protein they must properly and specifically combine the vegetables they eat. Francis Moore Lappé, who helped popularize the myth that vegetables must be properly combined in order to obtain complete protein in her 1971 book, *Diet for a Small Planet*, has admitted this premise was incorrect. Because of the enormous amount of research done recently on this topic, nearly every expert now agrees it is not necessary to "complement your proteins." And you don't have to consume foods from all the food groups at each meal. In fact, that would be a *bad* way to combine foods. In my book *Total Health Makeover*, I devoted an entire chapter to food combining. It is a way of eating that I really believe in, but I also believe that it is more important to get good food into children, in whatever combination they will eat it. Interestingly enough, children are often natural food combiners and will eat this way on their own. Refer to the food-combining chart on page 302-303 for the most efficient food combining.

The American meat-eating habit is killing us and it's not even necessary for protein! Bad cholesterol (low-density lipoproteins, or LDLs) in the diet comes exclusively from animal products. Cholesterol-clogged arteries are the main cause of about 50 percent of American deaths from heart disease and strokes. Vegetarians rarely have problems related to cholesterol. As Neal Barnard, M.D., president of the Physicians Committee for Responsible Medicine, said, "The beef industry has contributed to more American deaths than all the wars of this century, all natural disasters, and all automobile accidents combined."

Did you ever wonder where the flavor in meat comes from? Well, the flavor we taste in meat comes from the blood and uric acid (nitrogenous waste) within its flesh and other tissues. Yikes! I am sure that's why after twenty-two years of not eating meat, I cannot stand the smell of meat cooking—all that burning flesh! The uric acid is extremely taxing to our bodies; our liver and kidneys have to work overtime to break down the toxins in uric acid. We derive pleasure from one of the most dangerous elements of meat. It is a sad fact that Americans have grown up thinking that eating meat is required to receive our protein and proper nourishment. The popularity of meat is one of the biggest factors responsible for the deterioration of the health of Americans.

The concentration of pesticides found in meat is as much as ten times that of grains, fruits, and vegetables. Chemical and pesticide accumulation in the body is a serious matter. The higher the level a body consumes and stores, the higher the risk of cancer and liver failure. It is also not generally known by the public that cancer growths in animals are quite common. The butcher cuts these out at the slaughterhouse or supermarket before the meat is sold to the consumer. There is a vicious cycle that continues in the meat industry. Cattle and poultry become more and more immune to the drugs they are given to control their diseases, so it becomes necessary to develop even stronger and more deadly drugs and poisons.

Aside from drugs, disease, growths, and cancer, think about the unhygienic nature of dead animals. When meat is butchered at the slaughterhouse, meat inspectors are forced to work extremely fast. They have only seconds to check inside the dead animal for grubs, parasites, abscesses, and disease. Meat inspectors must inspect on average 300 carcasses an hour. That's only twelve seconds per carcass! Even if meat were raised organically and later butchered and prepared in the most pristine conditions, it would still be a problem for us because the human digestive system is simply not designed to eat meat. The structures of our skin, teeth, stomach, and bowels, and the length of our digestive system, are all typical of vegetarian animals.

> Half the antibiotics used in this country are used on farms. Whole flocks and herds are doused with antibiotics, often to compensate for poor conditions on the farm. Products label "antibiotic-free" refers to the time of slaughter, and not necessarily production. Buy meat from organic food producers instead.
>
> Dr. Patty Lieberman,
> Center for Science in the
> Public Interest

All animal products contain zero fiber. The lack of fiber in meat, dairy, and eggs makes them rot in the colon, causing constipation, body odor, and colon problems. (Have you ever smelled the breath of someone on a high protein–low carbohydrate diet?) It is the fiber found only in plants that acts as an "intestinal broom" to keep our colons clean and functioning efficiently.

The fast food and meat-packing industries are quite powerful and have great influence on Capitol Hill. That is why efforts to stop the dangerous and questionable practices in both industries are usually thwarted. The Physicians Committee for Responsible Medicine (PCRM) is one group that has been pressuring the U.S. government to make a greater effort to protect its citizens from diseases like mad-cow, hoof-and-mouth, and Creutzfeldt-Jakob disease (CJD), which is the mad-cow equivalent in humans. These diseases are believed to spread as a result of feeding contaminated meat and bonemeal to uncontaminated animals, as well as through combining contaminated products.

"Our government has been frighteningly slow to react to the very real threat of CJD in America," says PCRM president Neal D. Barnard, M.D. "The protective measures taken so far are grossly insufficient. We should learn from Europe's mistakes and implement tough precautionary measures now, before it's too late."

Dr. Barnard adds, "There is no restriction on the use of blood and blood products, gelatin, milk, and milk products in feeds. There are no limits on the use of pig or horse remains in feeds, due to an exception in the 1997 ban. There are no limits on the 'recycling' of beef or other meat products in the form of garbage from restaurants or other institutions for use in animal feeds. Ruminant remains can be fed to poultry, and in turn, poultry feces and litter are routinely used in cattle feed.

"Meat is simply a risky product," says Dr. Barnard. "And it's not just CJD that people need to worry about: Heart disease, colon cancer, diabetes, hypertension, and many other dangerous diseases—not to mention foodborne illnesses—would be greatly diminished by avoiding meat entirely."

Eating meat is not only detrimental to our bodies; it's also bad for our environment. It always amazes me that schools take the time to teach children about the effects of pollution on our environment, but never seem to mention that animal agriculture in the U.S. is one of the largest polluters and consumers of energy. It takes 2,500 gallons of water to produce one pound of beef, and three pounds of grain to make one Quarter Pounder. Add to this the additional loss of thirty-five pounds of topsoil, when it takes 500 years to make one inch! This is one of the least efficient uses of our food and natural resources. The meat industry is not only harmful to our health and environment, but also to our global society. Anthropologists and agricultural experts have complained for years that meat cultivation is the least efficient choice for feeding the population at large, yet over 50 percent of the world's grain and over 70 percent of U.S. grain is grown to feed livestock. One of the most embarrassing contradictions we see in the world today is that an unprecedented percentage of the world (especially the Western world) is obese and overweight, yet malnutrition continues to grow worldwide. Twenty million people starve to death every year. It's been estimated that if meat consumption were cut by just 10 percent, the world's food resources would increase enough to feed 100 million people. By switching your family's standard American diet (meat and dairy based) to a diet based primarily on plant foods, you improve your chances of living a long, healthy life, and help improve the ecological balance of our planet.

Dairy

I know I am going out on a limb with this one, but there is no way I cannot share the information I have learned about dairy products with parents who are concerned about their children's health. I am asking you to read the facts and open your mind. For twenty-two years I have been studying the effects of dairy on the human body. I know from my own family's experiences and the experiences of families who visit (marilu.com) my Web site that dairy does not always do a body good.

What is the first food a doctor or allergist will tell you to remove from your diet if you are congested or are having problems digesting? DAIRY! Cow's milk and other dairy products are always at the top of the list as the leading cause of food allergies. These allergies most commonly surface in the form of diarrhea, fatigue, constipation, irritability, and respiratory problems. However, these symptoms almost always disappear after dairy is removed from a child's diet. Even the dairy industry recognizes that milk products need a pill to help them become digested properly. As my son said after watching a commercial for Lactaid, "Why would anyone want to take a pill to be able to eat something? Why don't they just not eat dairy in the first place?"

Although the reputation of cow's milk is plummeting quickly in the United States, infants, children, teenagers, adults, and senior citizens still consume plenty of it along with other dairy products like cheese, butter, and yogurt. We see images of strong, healthy athletes and beautiful models and actors telling us how strong and healthy milk will make us. For many of us it was our first food, since many infants skip breast-feeding altogether. But cow's milk used in formula is considered the reason why fatty streaks and cholesterol accumulations are found in infants as young as nine months old. We all recognize that breast-feeding is a much better choice than bottle-feeding with cow's milk formula. But what about when a child moves on to solid foods? Is cow's milk a good choice for a growing toddler or child?

Could there be anything wrong with milk? We all grew up with this very popular beverage, and many still feel comforted by it. Americans are usually surprised to find out that most people on this planet have never even had one glass of milk in their lives, and if they did, most would get very sick. Since we were kids, we have been led to believe that milk is a perfect food. There have now been many studies done proving the opposite. Dairy products play a major role in the development of allergies, sleep disorders, kidney stones, mucus production, hemoglobin loss, depression, mood swings, irritability, and even arthritis in infants and children.

Have you ever wondered what the difference is between the composition of cow's milk and human breast milk? They are quite different. In fact, the milk of every species of mammal is unique. Each is perfectly designed to develop its own particular offspring most efficiently. Cow's milk is much richer in protein than human milk, four times, in fact, and has five to seven times the mineral content. You might say, "Great! Even better!" But it is too much protein and too much mineral content for humans, and it is extremely deficient in the essential fatty acids that are abundant in human milk, which has six to ten more. Cow's milk is considerably deficient in linolenic acid, and skimmed cow's milk has none. These fatty acids are the building blocks for neurological development and delicate neuromuscular control in humans.

Cow's milk is designed to build massive skeletal and muscle tissue. As I am always saying, "Milk is specifically designed to turn a 45-pound calf into a 300-pound cow in six to eight months." (In other words, cow's milk is great if you want your baby to grow up to do a lot of plowing or grazing!) It is also much higher in sodium, fat, and phosphorous and much lower in potassium than human breast milk. Cow's milk protein is mostly casein, while the protein of human breast milk is mostly lactalbumin. This is far easier for an infant to digest.

Cow's milk is simply NOT designed for humans. This should come as no surprise, since cows are genetically distant from humans. One British study revealed that breast-fed babies had, on the average, IQ scores that were ten points higher than babies nursed with cow's milk–based formula. Human breast milk is the only food that is perfectly designed for the building of infant brain tissue. Other studies have found significant neurological disorders in babies raised solely on cow's milk. Similar neurological disorders were even found in adults who had subsisted for an extended time entirely on cow's milk through a gastric feeding tube. In both groups, infants and adults, the disorders disappeared when they returned to a diet that contained the essential fatty acids that are missing in cow's milk. This argument against dairy would be strong enough even if cow's milk were pure. But it no longer is pure. In fact, it is far from it.

The milk we grew up with no longer exists. Fifty years ago, the average cow from the top dairy companies produced an average of 2,000 pounds of milk per year. Today, the average cow produces about 50,000 pounds per year because of steroids, hormone therapy, and force-feeding plans. Because of these added bovine growth hormones, or BGH, there's a marked increase in mastitis, which then requires antibiotic therapy. So we end up with a product that lacks the fatty acids essential for brain tissue growth and contains a significant amount of growth hormones and antibiotics. Why in the world would we want this poison in our child's digestive system?

There's more. Blood is found in nearly all cow's milk. The USDA actually allows one-thirtieth of an ounce of white blood cells (better known as pus cells) per milliliter of milk. FDA inspectors also use very loose standards. They use a detection method that uncovers only two of the thirty or so drugs found in milk. Infections under cow's udders is common. These require ointments and antibiotics. Penicillin, one of the antibiotics used, is commonly found in samples of cow's milk. The insulinlike growth factor IGF-I, found in cow's milk, has been associated with breast, prostate, colon, and lung cancer. It has been confirmed in hundreds of studies that cow's milk and dairy products have been linked to heart disease. In many studies, milk and milk products were found to have a higher connection to heart disease than even heavy animal meats such as beef and pork. Greenland Eskimos have a high fat, high protein diet, yet have a very low incidence of heart disease. This is probably due to the fact that they rarely drink milk.

Several studies have concluded that the bovine serum albumin is the milk protein responsible for the onset of diabetes. Many infant formulas in industrialized countries are cow's milk based, making cow's milk the first foreign protein that enters an infant's digestive system in industrialized countries like the United States. Antibodies to bovine casein are present in over a third of IDDM (insulin-dependent diabetes mellitus) patients. So infants who drink well-known commercial formulas in industrialized countries could be starting on a road to diabetes as early as one week old. In fact, exposure to dairy products and high milk consumption in childhood may increase the risk of a child's developing juvenile diabetes. In an issue of *Diabetes Care* in 1994, one researcher claimed, based on twenty well-documented studies, that the link between milk and juvenile diabetes is "very solid."

Chronic ear infections that afflict up to 40 percent of children under the age of six are caused primarily by milk allergies. Less frequent ear infections during childhood are also associated with cow's milk allergies. When a child has chronic ear infections, an increasing number of doctors today recommend the elimination of milk and other dairy products from the child's diet for about thirty days. This almost always clears up chronic ear infections. Ear infections are rarely seen among children who don't consume any cow's milk or other dairy products.

I recently eliminated all dairy from my children's diet. I have three boys, and they had constant ear infections. This had been going on for years and years with rounds and rounds of antibiotics. I had questioned my pediatrician about dairy and she told me, "It isn't the dairy; we would have known by now." I finally decided to take their health into my own hands, and after extensive reading, I decided to take them completely off dairy. I am totally amazed at how cooperative they have been. They are so tired of being sick that they are willing to try anything! I told them it is an experiment that we will try for 2 to 3 months to see if they feel better. My oldest told me that he no longer feels that icky stuff in the back of his throat. I didn't even know he had it. When I questioned him about it, he told me he used to have it all the time and now it is gone.—DEBRA McCLOSKEY, MARILU.COM

In the past, cow's milk was considered by most doctors to be very desirable for the growth of a child. This has changed. The majority of doctors now agree that cow's milk contributes to an exhaustive list of health problems in children.

Dairy products contains twenty-five different proteins that are difficult for an adult to digest, and more so an infant or small child. Most gastrointestinal, skin, respiratory, behavioral, and blood disorders are dairy related. The incidence of crib death is higher when the baby or breast-feeding mother consumes dairy products. Dairy products have been linked to Hodgkin's disease, which is cancer of the immune system.

Colic is strongly linked to dairy products. Many pediatricians today recommend eliminating milk and dairy products for babies with colic. It is usually the result of an allergic reaction. As I stated earlier, there's a strong link between cow's milk and allergies, and practically no connection between allergies and human breast milk when the mother is dairy free; however, allergies are frequently found in breast-fed babies when the mother consumed dairy products during the months of breast-feeding.

> Cow's milk contains five and a half times more toxic pesticides than plant foods.

Significant improvements have been found in children with asthma after they gave up dairy products. Children with skin disorders such as eczema and dermatitis usually find relief after giving up dairy products, as well.

Eczema is almost always connected to food allergies and 9 times out of 10 that allergy is dairy. I have 2 friends who both struggled with eczema for years and no amount of medication seemed to make a difference. It wasn't until they gave up dairy that it cleared up for the first time in years.

—STEPHANIE HAYES, MARILU.COM

Bed-wetting has also been linked to cow's milk and dairy. In fact, "Does your child wet his bed?" is one of the first questions I ask parents when they tell me their child may have a problem with dairy. Trying to "break down" dairy also puts an unnecessary strain on the kidneys. It is also well known that allergies associated with dairy can cause the bladder to become inflamed, enlarged, and sensitive, creating a feeling of fullness, which leads to bed-wetting, and if that's not enough, dairy has also been known to cause constipation. If your child suffers from bedwetting or chronic constipation, I urge you to reconsider dairy products.

I'm the mother of three children ages 5, 2½, and 1. I tried to make sure that their diets were healthy and full of variety that included a lot of dairy for growing bones! When my middle child stopped nursing, I switched him to whole milk, and he was constipated. I thought he would grow out of it or his body would adjust. He loved milk and cheese, so I tried to adjust the entire rest of his diet accordingly. The poor child would be lying on my lap crying with constipation. I'd give him infant suppositories almost daily. With all the dairy (supposedly calcium) he was taking, he still broke his leg twice! My youngest child always had a runny nose, eyes, and mouth. We nicknamed him "goo-boy." You couldn't pick him up without a tissue. I thought it was teething. As soon as the dairy was gone, so was the "goo." I don't know what took me so long to get it. The final factor was

A recent study linked cow's milk consumption to chronic constipation in children. Researchers suggest that milk consumption resulted in perianal sores and severe pain on defecation, leading to constipation.

The Cancer Project

reading Total Health Makeover *and discovering better sources for calcium. We verified it was the dairy after he had some cheese at his grandparents'. The next day, the boys were a mess again. I wish I hadn't been so brain-washed before. My children are healthy and dairy free.*—WENDY K., OHIO

Vomiting, bloating, constipation and/or diarrhea also are often eliminated when children give up dairy products. It depends on the child. Instead of giving your children products such as Pepto-Bismol when they have diarrhea, try eliminating dairy products. Dairy products have also been linked to mood swings, depression, and irritability. I wonder how many kids out there are taking large doses of Ritalin when the problem is simply diet.

The type of calcium in dairy products can actually inhibit the absorption of iron. Rectal bleeding in infancy, which also causes iron loss, has been directly linked to cow's milk. Nearly every case of infant rectal bleeding disappeared after a switch was made to a formula free of cow's milk. It has been found in 30 percent of infants that blood loss in the intestinal tract comes from a reaction to cow's milk proteins. Most people assume that an infant gets more minerals from cow's milk; yet iron deficiency is one of the many consequences of drinking formula containing cow's milk because it leads to intestinal bleeding, which ultimately can lower an infant's hemoglobin count. What often follows is weakness, depression, and irritability. Iron deficiency is one of the most prevalent nutritional problems of children in the United States. Iron deficiency in infancy has been linked to lower IQ scores later in life. Iron deficiency and anemia have also been linked to shortened attention span, irritability, and fatigue. Consequently, anemic children tend to do poorly on vocabulary, reading, and other tests.

I have been begging people for years to rethink the whole dairy issue. Of the ten steps I took to change my health, I can honestly say that giving up dairy was the most difficult for me to do, but definitely the step that most improved my health and the health of my family.

Fat

Fat is a big issue with kids and adults. It is one of the most misunderstood aspects of diet and nutrition, and one of the most important. Logically it would seem that the trick to avoid *getting* fat is to avoid *eating* fat. When parents are concerned about their child being overweight, they usually try to eliminate or severely limit the fat in their child's diet. Also, because there is so much talk in the media linking fat with cholesterol and heart disease, it is commonly assumed that avoidance of fat is the key to both a healthy heart *and* a slim body. Well, conquering fat is not that simple. To begin with, we don't want to conquer fat completely. We need *some* fat in our diet. It's necessary. Like carbohydrates and protein, fat is an important source of energy. In fact, fat is the most concentrated source of energy in the diet. It provides nine calories per gram, compared with only four calories per gram from either carbohydrates or protein. Fats are composed mostly of the same three elements as carbohydrates (carbon, hydrogen, and oxygen). However, fats have more carbon and hydrogen and less oxygen, thus supplying the higher fuel value of nine calories per gram. Fat is a particularly important source of calories for infants and young children; 50 percent of the calories in human breast milk come from fat. It supplies essential fatty acids, such as linoleic and linolenic acids, which, once again, are especially important to children for proper growth. Fat insulates you against cold weather and acts as a shock absorber for your bones and internal organs like your heart and kidneys. Without fat, we're not able to absorb fat-soluble vitamins like A, D, E, and K. Often, when a woman's fat level drops low enough, she stops ovulating. Fat is also necessary for healthy hair and skin. Now, before you rush out with the kids for vanilla shakes and double bacon cheeseburgers, READ ON!

It's extremely important to know how much fat you should include in your kids' diet and which kinds of fats are acceptable. Fat is divided into two major categories: saturated, or "bad" fats, and unsaturated, or "good" fats (which can be mono or poly). Red meat, butter, cheese, ice cream, mayonnaise, cookies, and cake are all examples of foods containing bad fat. For the most part, saturated fats occur almost exclusively in animal products (the exceptions are coconut oil and palm oil), while unsaturated fats come from plant or fish sources (like olives, soybeans, corn, sardines, and salmon). Saturated fats are generally solid at room temperature and unsaturated fats are usually liquid at room temperature. Saturated fats can raise your cholesterol levels (especially LDL, the "bad cholesterol") and increase your risk of heart disease. Unsaturated fats (both mono- and polyunsaturated) can help lower cholesterol levels and reduce your risk of heart disease.

Okay, now this all makes sense. All you have to do is eliminate saturated fats from your family's diet and add, in moderation, healthy unsaturated fats, right? Well . . . not so fast. Here is where this all gets complicated. Fat classification is determined not by whether it comes from a plant or animal source, but by its chemical structure and the amount of hydrogen atoms that are attached to it. Saturated fats are completely full of hydrogen atoms. They cannot accept additional hydrogen atoms, hence the name "saturated." Monounsaturated and polyunsaturated fats are missing hydrogen atoms in places in their molecular structure. Unsaturated fats are classified based on the number of missing hydrogen atoms in their molecular structure—mono (can accept one hydrogen atom) or poly (can accept more than one hydrogen atom). Except for fish, which contains polyunsaturated fat, all other mono and poly fat come from plant sources.

Here is the most interesting (and scary) part. Scientists and food manufacturers have found a way to make unsaturated fats act like saturated fats. They bombard the unsaturated fat molecules with hydrogen, and those places that were once missing hydrogen in their molecular structure now have hydrogen. And PRESTO! You now have a man-made saturated fat—also known as a trans fatty acid. The process is called hydrogenation. There are a lot of benefits to this for the food processors, definitely *not* for us. Hydrogenation increases the stability of a fat or oil, which is important in cooking and extending a product's shelf life. (Food processors sure do love to extend their products' shelf life, don't they?) Hydrogenation is also used to convert liquid oils to a semisolid form because this man-made saturated fat now behaves just like saturated fat (solid at room temperature). For example, vegetable oils are often hydrogenated to produce shortenings or margarines. The more hydrogen, the harder the oil will be at room temperature.

Unsaturated fats, especially polyunsaturated fats, have a tendency to break down when exposed to air and quickly develop an offensive flavor and odor. Adding hydrogen molecules makes the fatty acids more stable and resistant to oxidation. This is especially important for fats used in deep-frying. Hydrogenation is also great for making the texture of the food product containing the fat more desirable. The firmness and spreadability of margarines, flakiness of pie crust, and creaminess of puddings all depend on how much hydrogenation is used.

Along with all of these benefits, the food processors can also claim to be selling a healthier product because "it's from a vegetable source, so it's not that bad for you." And for many years, we believed this. The problem is that our bodies can't tell the difference between the real saturated fats and the man-made saturated fats—trans fatty acids. The trans fatty acids can raise blood cholesterol the same way the real saturated fats do. They may even be worse for you and your children than the saturated fats we've done our best to avoid most of our lives. The scariest part of all is that these hydrogenated oils seem to be used in everything! You can easily spot trans fats in food products by looking for the words "partially hydrogenated" or "hydrogenated" in the list of ingredients.

I want to say a few things about cholesterol because so many people are worried about it. Cholesterol is different from saturated or unsaturated fat. It is necessary in the making of cell walls and hormones. It would be fine if you never consumed any foods containing cholesterol because your body makes more than double the supply you need. It is the excess cholesterol, especially LDL, in the blood that leads to clogged arteries, but the main culprit is more likely to be saturated fats and the trans fatty acids we were just talking about, more than cholesterol itself. My advice is to avoid all three. Food from a plant source does not have any cholesterol (it is made in the liver of animals). As long as you limit your consumption of animal products, you won't have to worry about extra cholesterol.

All fats, whether saturated, unsaturated, or trans fat, have the same number of calories (nine calories per gram). Olive oil (which is considered to be good for your heart) has the same amount of calories as butter (a potentially artery-clogging killer). Stick with totally unhydrogenated unsaturated fats, and then only in moderation! You have to be very careful here because trans fatty acids are hidden in nearly every commercially prepared food on the market that contains fat. The food labeling laws do not require food processors to list the quantities of trans fatty acids in any food. That means that food products that claim to have no cholesterol (because they contain no naturally saturated fats) can actually be *loaded* with trans fat while claiming to contain only "100 percent vegetable oil." That's why you have to check the list of ingredients to see if whatever the vegetable oil used is partially or completely hydrogenated. I guarantee you won't see any mention of trans fat on there. As far as partially hydrogenated is concerned, I would avoid ANY hydrogenation. A hydrogenated vegetable oil is labeled "partial" whether it's been 75 percent hydrogenated or 20 percent hydrogenated.

During the 1980s, when there was a lot of bad press about saturated animal fats, the fast food companies announced that they were switching from animal fat to 100 percent vegetable oil. What kind of vegetable oil? You guessed it, partially *hydrogenated* vegetable oil! Now the fries are just as bad for your heart as the burger, maybe worse! I know that for some of you this is an eye-opener. And you may even feel discouraged about the daunting task of throwing out half the items in your refrigerator and cupboard, but trust me, it's worth it for you and your kids. The most important things to look for when shopping, and avoid completely, are foods with vegetable shortening and partially hydrogenated oils. Avoid deep-fried foods, especially in fast food restaurants. Better yet, simply avoid fast food restaurants altogether. At home and when dining out, substitute olive oil or canola oil for butter, margarine, or shortening.

Caffeine

When kids consume a lot of candy and soft drinks, sugar is not the only problem. One study found that the average child consumed over 300 milligrams of caffeine daily from colas, candy, and chocolate. That's equivalent to nearly five cups of coffee! We adults know the effect caffeine has on our system. It gives us a quick energy burst, then drops us off a cliff, and we're forced to get through our day with no vitality. That is why we often feel tired and irritable at work during the afternoon. It's no wonder that children become so cranky an hour or so after having chocolate, colas, and other soft drinks. They are forced to do schoolwork and attend to other responsibilities when all they really want is a nap.

Most parents wouldn't think of giving their child a cup of coffee, but think nothing of allowing them to drink several cans of soda full of caffeine and sugar. As with sugar, many experts believe that large doses of caffeine can cause children to behave as though they have hyperactive disorders. Children get the same buzz we adults get from a cup of coffee, but it is worse for children because their bodies are so much smaller. But that's not all. According to a 1994 Harvard study, soda consumption increases the risk of bone fracture because caffeine leaches small amounts of calcium from the bones.

Have you ever wondered why caffeine is added to soft drinks? According to the National Soft Drink Association, the caffeine is added for the taste, not the buzz. If that were the case, one would assume that kids could easily tell the difference between sodas with or without caffeine. Well, *Consumer Reports* did a nationwide taste test with over 400 middle-school children who tasted unmarked samples of Mountain Dew and the caffeine-free version sold in Canada. They were also given Sunkist Orange and its caffeine-free equivalent. The children were asked to pick the better-tasting soda, and each test was done six times to see if a child could consistently pick the same sample. Eighty percent of the kids chose inconsistently between the two. In other words, they were unable to taste the difference between the caffeinated and uncaffeinated drinks. Our children are getting caffeine unnecessarily. Could the major soft drink companies be adding caffeine just to get kids hooked on caffeine?

Another problem is that, under current Food and Drug Administration standards, products are not required to reveal the exact amount of caffeine they contain. Children who drink soft drinks of any kind are probably getting more caffeine than we realize. My advice is to remove all sugar-sweetened soft drinks from your home, whether or not they are caffeinated or sugar-sweetened or Nutrasweetened. Try 100 percent fruit juice Knudsen Spritzers if your kids want something like a soda. Or better yet, stick to 100 percent fruit juice diluted with water.

Chemicals

Are food additives really all that dangerous for our kids? There are over 3,000 hidden chemicals in our food, and the average American consumes over one pound of food additives a year. Additives such as dyes, nitrates, emulsifiers, fillers, tenderizers, waxers, texturizers, MSG, antibiotics, and even "tasty" things like antifreeze are used to preserve and enhance flavor, texture, and appearance in our everyday foods. A brief list of the most common problems associated with many of these 3,000 additives includes tumors and serious side effects in lab animals; heart, lung, and kidney disease; birth defects; nausea and vomiting; dangerous levels of toxicity (in other words, poison); and carcinogens.

An example of a food that many people assume is safe is ice cream. Aside from the fact that it contains dairy (you already know how I feel about dairy!), ice cream is deadly for other reasons. Many ice creams contain diethyl glucol, which is also used in antifreeze and paint removers. Other substances found in ice cream are piperonal (also used to exterminate lice), some cherry flavorings (also used in rubber dyes and plastics), pineapple flavorings (also used to clean textiles and leather), nut flavorings (used in rubber cement), and the list goes on. The amazing thing is that the food manufacturers are not required to list these chemicals by their real names, like ethyl acetate or amyl acetate, on the label. They can simply say it's banana flavoring. That's why labels that appear to be somewhat safe are actually hiding many harmful substances and chemicals.

Of course, the best way to avoid these dangers is to eat as many natural whole foods as possible. The more processing involved, the more likely that product will contain chemicals and additives. In a five-year study from 1979 to 1984, Dr. Stephen Schoenthaler organized a diet plan for the New York City School system. Working with the food supervisors for 800,000 pupils, they removed all of the artificial colors, flavors, sugars, and additives from the breakfast and lunch cafeteria menus. They substituted natural whole grains, fruits, and vegetables for the entire five-year period. During those years, the average achievement test score went from a below average of 39 to an above average of 52. After the project was over and the menus returned to typical American junk food, full of additives and chemicals, the average student's test scores dropped to the low scores that were posted before the experiment.

I went to a symposium recently on women's health issues conducted by six eminent physicians. At one point, during a lecture on children and chemicals, one of the doctors said that because of the high content of nitrates found in today's American hot dogs, a child who consumes an average of six or more hot dogs a week would ingest a level of nitrates that would put him beyond what is considered a dangerous risk for cancer later in life. One woman raised her hand and said, "Well, how many hot dogs can I safely serve my kids a week?" And I shouted out, "How about NONE!" What was she trying to find out—how many she could give them to be just under the cancer level? What a ridiculous question. But I don't really blame her. I think that is the way many people think about diet and nutrition for themselves and their kids today. It's like Jerry Seinfeld's line about the silly concept of *extra strength* painkillers. He says, "Let's figure out the amount of Excedrin that will kill us, and then give us just a little less." I think the biggest problem in this country is that people do not make the connection between what they eat, how they feel, and how it affects their health. And we're doing it to our kids over and over again under the guise of giving them treats and not wanting to look as if we're not loving, generous parents. We buy big, colorful candies instead of fruits and raisins. We give our kids what they want, not what is best for them.

3

Family Attitudes

Avoiding Food as a Comfort, Reward, or Punishment

We have looked at some of the facts about our children's health today, and what we are feeding their little bodies. But now let's look at an issue that is perhaps more important—what are we feeding their impressionable little minds? What examples are we setting with our own behavior and attitudes toward food that could be shaping *their* way of thinking about it? What are they learning from us (which we probably learned from our parents) that may be causing some of the health problems that are so common today? We know that good nutrition starts at home, and we will focus on the specifics of a wholesome, natural way of eating in the next few chapters. But first, let's talk about a sensible way of "thinking" about food. Practically all of us have grown up associating food with reward and punishment. We have all heard statements like "Eat your vegetables, or you won't get dessert" or "Finish what's on your plate, and I'll give you more" or "If you go to your piano lesson, I'll take you out for ice cream." Every kid in my neighborhood associated doctors and getting sick with a big reward. We all prayed for a tonsillectomy because of rumors of all-you-can-eat ice cream.

As a kid, I actually looked forward to going to the doctor. My mother used to drive us way outside the city limits of Chicago to go to our family physician, Dr. Midgley. His office was out in farm country, which at that time was only about forty minutes north of Chicago. That's barely considered a suburb by today's standards, but back then it felt like we were driving to Nebraska. It was one of those special times when we got to see cows, pigs, horses, and even silos. All of my friends went to doctors in the city, so I knew it was odd that we would drive so far to go to a country doctor. Even back then, at age ten, I thought it was because my mother had an innocent crush on Dr. Midgley. (Now that I'm older and wiser, I'm *sure* that was the reason!)

After getting examined, all of us kids would line up to get our booster shot. The thing I remember most was that after the shot, we would each get a sucker, but unfortunately, Dr. Midgley never had enough RED ones. So I, of course, always wanted to be the first kid in line, so I would be first to pick out a sucker. If there was only one red one, that baby was *mine*. What a wonderful feeling it was to lift up that bright red sucker to my mouth with my prizewinning sore shoulder.

This was a big deal to me. I vividly remember the little white box that held the suckers. In fact, I remember the sucker box better than I remember Dr. Midgley. Anyway, the point I'm trying to make here is that this is what adults did, and still do, to keep kids in line. The pain of getting a shot was relieved by the pleasure of getting to eat a sucker. Food (sweets in particular) become the cure-all, the Band-Aid, the device used to relieve all of our suffering, and of course, a tool to persuade. If you skin your knee, you get a cookie. If you get an A on a math test, you go out for a hot fudge sundae. Food is not regarded as it should be, what it truly is—life sustenance. I know that sounds like a boring way to look at food, but believe me, when you begin to think of it as life's nutrition and not as some naughty treat or Band-Aid for disappointment, that's when food becomes most exciting. Sitting down and eating together as a family always has been, and should remain, one of life's great pleasures. But food too often is used as a reward/punishment tool. Because of this, it's become part of our everyday pain-comfort cycle. Whenever our feelings are hurt, or we have a setback at school or work, we immediately turn to the comfort of food. Any of life's bumps, pains, or suffering gets rewarded, comforted, or soothed by having some kind of treat. You break up with your boyfriend, and there you are knocking back a quart of Häagen-Dazs. We turn to food to celebrate our victories in life, too. "I just got a big bonus at work today, so I'm treating all of you to dinner." Unfortunately, for many people, that hot fudge sundae or little red sucker is now a bottle of scotch and/or a pack of cigarettes.

My parents were wonderful, but they unknowingly helped me develop some bad eating habits. With six kids in my family, competition for food was fierce. It was essential for survival to load up your plate early to get your fair share—and a little bit more, if you could get away with it. However, my father, the chairman of the Clean Plate Club, had zero tolerance for wasted food. He would say, "Finish that first, and then I'll give you more." Once an item made it to our plate, we had better finish it. It was like trying to get your money's worth at an all-you-can-eat buffet every day, but getting fined for not finishing "everything." As a child, I never learned how to stop eating when I was full; I learned to stop when my plate was *empty*. That attitude creates a relationship with food in which fullness, and not your body's natural instinct to stop, is associated with "finishing." It took me years of struggling with my weight and then learning about nutrition and health before I found my body's true appetite.

But I am one of the lucky ones. If left to develop, this pattern of not listening to your body's natural appetite can begin a cycle that starts in childhood and can take years, even a lifetime, to reverse. It's hard to find a home or school in America where this food-reward-punishment syndrome isn't practiced. (And then we wonder why we have so much child obesity and behavioral problems in school.)

So what can we do? How do we break this cycle? How do we keep from passing on from generation to generation the things that grown-ups did to us as kids? The first step toward breaking this cycle of destructive behavior is to become aware of it. We must realize that years of filling our guts with pleasure food to relieve pain will only cause a whole new pain—the pain of having to lose a lot of weight or having to recover from the toxicity caused by years of junk food. Or, more important, the pain of a lower self-esteem. And after becoming aware of it, we have to stop relieving our child's pain with comfort food or stop rewarding our child's accomplishments with pleasure food. How about trying to establish some kind of nonfood prize to reward a child? I'm not saying you shouldn't go out to dinner to celebrate with your kids; I'm just saying that if your child needs comfort or a reward, avoid using food or treats. Instead, try rewarding or comforting with some form of attention. You may be surprised to find that reading a book together or playing a game means more than a hot fudge sundae. If your son's soccer team wins, instead of taking them to a drive-thru, take them to a driving range (or miniature golf!). Buy a toy, take a walk together, or, best of all, simply tell them you're proud. There are so many possibilities. Be creative, but don't involve food. Actually, the best lesson they could learn is that the accomplishment is the reward itself. And when a child fails at something or gets bruised emotionally or physically, don't reach for the cookie jar. Instead, think of a more personal, less destructive way to comfort her. Sometimes the best choice you can make for her is to let her face her disappointment without any anesthetic. This will strengthen her character and better prepare her for the real world.

Besides using food as a comfort, punishment, or reward, consider other negative behavioral patterns you may be guilty of that may be rubbing off on your kids. What are your own health habits? If you're the kind of parent who starts the day with a cup of coffee, sweet roll, and a cigarette for breakfast, what kind of message do you think that sends to your child? Children learn by example. If you have a good attitude about food and typically eat fresh fruits, vegetables, whole grains, and lean proteins, it will be a lot easier to teach your kids to be healthy, because you're healthy. If you smoke, drink, eat junk food, or your weight fluctuates wildly because of reducing pills or crazy diets, your child will learn from that, too, and will often develop a similar relationship with food.

I remember this one friend's daughter. She was getting dressed for her *third* birthday and didn't want to wear a dress because she thought it made her thighs look chubby. And I remember thinking, "Oh my gosh, if this is how she feels at three, what will she be like at twelve or sixteen?" And then I realized she was a Mini-Me version of her mom, who has similar dramas about her wardrobe. We have to watch what kind of message we are sending our children about diet and self-image. We are not going to get them to eat healthy if our relationship to food is so unnatural and self-conscious.

Breaking Your Own Family Cycle

Because kids are so impressionable and learn most things by example, the most decisive factor for your children's health is you guys, their parents. It is extremely important for parents to set a good example.

If you build it, they will come. That is really the main theme of this book—if you are not putting good, healthy, vibrant food into yourself every day, how do you expect to get it into your kids? You can't expect your children to eat wholesome foods if you're always snacking on potato chips and ice cream. If your refrigerator and cupboards are full of only junk food, laden with the "white foods"—sugar, fat, white flour, dairy, and chemicals—how do you expect them to get the message? But if you can stock your refrigerator with wholesome, healthy food, eventually your kids are going to eat it because that's what's available. A diet change for your children has to be a diet change for the whole family. (That includes you, too, Dad!) If a parent is allowed to eat candy and sweets in front of the children while they are forbidden, resentment and battles will almost always follow. It is also not a good idea to single out the overweight child. The most successful weight-loss programs for children are those that consistently involve the entire family. A healthy, natural, whole food diet is best, whether your child is obese or underweight. Whatever your children do in the outside world is difficult, or impossible, for you to control. But if you make an effort at home to give your kids the food and nutrition that will give them energy, balance, and a good attitude all day, eventually they are going to enjoy feeling good. And they are going to make a connection between what they eat and how they feel. And isn't that what we are trying to do here? We are trying to help our children be their strongest, happiest, and healthiest because we love them.

I think that what's important is truly believing that this is more than just a healthy way for them to eat. This is a lifesaving way for them to eat. By putting up with the "this tastes bad" or "this tastes funny" until they (and we) get used to the new textures and tastes, we are giving them a longer, healthier, and more productive life. Hats off to you who have gotten your kids eating and living healthy. The best parents are those who do what's best for the kids, not what's easiest for the parents!—Natasha M. Hope, Utah

Portion Size Increase

"Super Size," "All-you-can-eat," "Big Gulp," "Jumbo Jack." These days, it seems the best way to lure customers is to give them a lot more than they actually need. How many times have you said to yourself, "Gee, I really don't need the Super-Colossal-Mucho-Grande size, but it's such a *bargain*"? People will choose a restaurant because of its reputation for huge portions. Being able to "supersize" a fast food meal is seen as a big bonus. I guess people want to make sure that under no circumstances should they ever be even a tiny bit hungry at the end of the meal. They say that people's number one fear in life is public speaking. But sometimes I think it's the fear of not being completely stuffed at the end of a meal. In my entire life, I have never heard anyone on the way home from a restaurant say, "Darn it! Why didn't I order more?" On the other hand, I've heard a thousand people (myself included) say, "Ooooooooohhhh! Why did I eat so much?" At least one person says it every time we go out.

My friends from Europe are always so surprised at how huge the portions are in the United States. There is no such thing as a doggie bag in other countries, unless, of course, the clientele is mostly American tourists. Sometimes I get the feeling that the rest of the world views Americans the same way we Americans view Las Vegas—flashy, excessive, greedy, and unhealthy. The funny thing is, I *like* Las Vegas. It's got the same kind of appeal that a wacky relative has at the family Christmas party. You know he's gonna do something outrageous. You just don't know what it will be.

During my teens, I was a waitress at a family vacation resort called Nippersink Manor near Lake Geneva, Wisconsin. It was very similar to the resort in the movie *Dirty Dancing*. (And I was exactly like Jennifer Grey!) Anyway, we would serve an average of 500 guests per meal. On some occasions, the meals were served all-you-can-eat buffet style instead of the usual menu service. The chef told me that on buffet days the kitchen had to prepare three times what they normally prepare because people will eat two to three times their usual amount when given no limit. That's why buffets are so dangerous for many people—because they often load up their plates while completely ignoring portion size. Oh, they'll have the standard six-ounce piece of fish, but they'll also have the six-ounce cut of prime rib, the six-ounce pork chop, three pieces of southern-fried chicken, and a slice of pepperoni pizza. And you know how they feel after that? Like having ice cream! On apple pie!! Why? Because they don't want to waste the opportunity! It was so funny to watch people's eyes light up when they would take their first stroll around the buffet table to carefully plan their "dining strategy." Most were thinking, "I guess I'm going to be here a while, so I'll need about three dozen napkins, my mail forwarded, and a pair of my dad's pants."

You would hear people at each table exchanging past buffet triumphs like they were adventure travelers swapping safari stories. I heard a guy say once, "I had a prime rib buffet at the Sands in Las Vegas back in '72. Because I was smart enough to skip the rolls and mashed potatoes, I was able to eat three cuts of prime rib and seventeen Alaskan king crab legs!" He said it as if he very cleverly outsmarted the casino.

I remember at one Nippersink buffet, I saw an obese woman perspiring and panting heavily as she and her husband were staggering out of the dining room and I said, "Are you okay? Should I call a doctor?" The husband laughed and said, "No, no, don't worry, dear. She just overate at the buffet again! We just love your buffets!"

Since my summers at Nippersink, I've learned that overeating like that can be triggered two ways, psychologically and/or physiologically. Food visibility and availability at a buffet table (or even from something like a colorful menu at Denny's) are powerful eating stimuli and are very hard for some people to resist. For others, the problem is more physiological. They suffer from glucose intolerance. In this situation, the body does not metabolize carbohydrates normally. In a healthy body, carbohydrates are converted to glucose and a normal blood glucose level is maintained despite excessive carbohydrates consumed. In the glucose intolerant, excess carbohydrates are rapidly converted to glucose, and the pancreas responds to this shift in blood sugar by secreting an excessive amount of insulin.

Normally, the job insulin does is to remove the glucose from the bloodstream and help it to enter the cells in the body. If this is done properly, the blood glucose level returns to the normal range regardless of the amount of carbohydrates consumed, which is what happens when a person doesn't have glucose intolerance. The excessive insulin in the body of the glucose intolerant is a problem because the cells in the body do not recognize the insulin, and the glucose does not get removed from the bloodstream. The result is an increase in blood insulin levels, which has an appetite-stimulating effect. The person is driven to eat more, and the cycle continues.

If this sounds like your child, consult a physician. Often she will recommend that the child spread the calories out by frequently eating a small amount of food

> Several studies have found that as kids get older, they tend to eat whatever portion size is put in front of them, ignoring internal cues that tell them they're full. Some experts believe that eating larger portions may be one of the reasons why one out of every five kids in the United States is overweight.
>
> *Healthy Kids,*
> *October/November 2000*

every few hours. Avoid too much time between meals or your child will be ravenous and very likely want to overeat. Don't, however, push a child to eat before he is a little hungry, either. It can be difficult finding the best interval between meals. It takes some trial and error and listening carefully to your child's appetite signals to find the best times to eat and the amount to have at each meal. Also, sticking with vegetable proteins (beans, legumes, and nuts) and complex carbohydrates is very important for the kids with glucose intolerance. Seriously avoid simple sugars and carbohydrates (processed white flour and sugar). Complex carbohydrates, on the other hand, are great because they leave the stomach more slowly than simple carbohydrates and help in blood glucose regulation. Complex carbohydrates contain fiber. Soluble fiber is especially beneficial for this condition.

So, how did our culture get so consumed with consumption? People often say things like "I'm going to pig out this weekend, but I'll make up for it on Monday." Unfortunately, the body doesn't recover from a pig-out session so easily. The saddest part of all this is that children grow up today thinking that supersizing and overindulgence are normal. According to a study reported in the January 2000 issue of the *Journal of the American Dietetic Association*, children as early as age five begin to eat based more on serving size, not appetite. Before five, however, the study showed that most kids ate according to appetite. This shows that kids adapt, against their natural instincts, to overeating.

A big question for all of us now is just what is a healthy serving size? We've been served Fred Flintstone–size portions for so long, we no longer know what "normal" is.

Then and Now Serving Sizes

Item	Then	Now
Popcorn	3 cups	16 cups
Soda	8 ounces	32 to 64 ounces
Fast food burger	2 ounces	6 ounces
Fast food French fries	4 ounces	12 ounces

How Big Is a Serving?

1 ounce of protein	Matchbox
3 ounces of protein	Deck of cards
8 ounces of protein	Small paperback book

Medium apple or orange	Tennis ball
Medium potato	Computer mouse
1 cup of lettuce	4 green leaves
1 slice of bread	Cassette tape
1 ounce of cheese	4 dice
1 cup of fruit	Baseball

What Medical Doctors Are Taught About Nutrition

*In medical school, there is no emphasis on nutrition at all, and there is no training for it. In my four years of medical school, there were only nine hours devoted to nutrition. And I don't mean semester hours, I mean nine hours total! I think that nutrition is as important as learning about anatomy. If you learned about nutrition early on, when you went into practice, whether as an obstetrician or a pediatrician or an internist, you could sit down with your patients, see what they eat, and work with them. I think you would avoid a lot of diseases that cost this country billions of dollars. Right now you're losing people that get sick, that can't go to work, can't function, so you get a loss of productivity in the workplace. Not to mention that medical economics is insane.—*PETER S. WALDSTEIN, M.D., F.A.A.P.

*In this culture we are very good at fixing what's already broken. Doctors are good at doing heart transplants and bypass surgeries. But when it comes to lifestyle diseases like cardiovascular disease, high cholesterol, kidney disease, and diabetes, Western medicine gets very low marks. We are not that good at prevention.—*TED PASTRICK, M.P.T.

Have you ever gone to the doctor knowing that something is wrong, only to be given a prescription for a drug? You take the drug, but the side effects from it kick in, and pretty soon you are worse off than you were before. Finally you remember an old wives' tale about avoiding certain foods for your original condition, and when you try it because you are desperate, it works. So you think, "Why didn't my doctor tell me this?" Do you want the answer? It's because most doctors don't make the connection between what we eat and how we feel.

Treating patients nutritionally can increase their life spans, prevent and often cure diseases, stop or alleviate most human suffering, and significantly lower medical costs. Yet, only recently have U.S. medical schools begun to integrate nutrition into bedside and case-based teaching. Twenty percent of deaths in the United States are directly attributed to improper diet and lack of exercise. Physicians know how to treat illnesses but know very little about how to prevent them.

This does make sense, in a way, because some doctors may perceive healthy eating and nutrition as a threat. The healthier we are, the less we need them. It's like the old saying "An apple a day keeps the doctor away." Well, some doctors simply don't want to know about apples, and they unconsciously don't want us to know about them, either. I am not talking about all doctors, of course. I am just saying that it is important to find a doctor who knows enough about nutrition to work *with* you in order to maintain good health for you and your family. I have always believed that we should pay doctors to keep us healthy and stop paying them if we get sick. That would improve the health of America!

The National Academy of Sciences conducted an extensive study of the current nutrition programs in U.S. medical schools in 1985 and updated it in 2000. Here are some of the conclusions and recommendations they made as a result of this study:

◆ The teaching of nutrition in most U.S. medical schools is inadequate. The committee recommends that U.S. medical schools examine the nutrition component of their curriculum and take steps to remedy the deficiencies.

◆ Nutrition is not taught as a separate subject in the majority of schools surveyed. Although some nutritional concepts are taught in conjunction with other courses, they are frequently not identified as such and their impact and importance are accordingly diminished.

◆ All students should be given a course, or its equivalent, in the fundamentals of nutrition during the same years in which other basic sciences are offered. These concepts should be reinforced during later clinical clerkships, as students see and experience the application of nutrition to patient care.

◆ More than half the medical schools surveyed by the committee teach less than twenty hours of nutrition, and 20 percent of them teach less than ten hours.

+ The committee's review of the National Medical Board examinations indicates there is an inequity in the distribution of nutrition topics among questions on the basic sciences and on various medical specialties. Certain aspects of nutrition were strongly emphasized, whereas others were ignored.

+ The resources available for teaching nutrition in medical schools are insufficient. Faculty members who teach the subject concur that nutrition textbooks, although plentiful, are inadequate to meet their instructional needs. Thus, they must prepare their own syllabi. In addition, those schools that lack an appropriate faculty member offer only a minimum amount of course work on nutrition.

"Diet plays perhaps the most important role in the prevention of heart disease." In a nationwide survey done in 1999, only 60 percent of the physicians who responded agreed with that statement. The key word here is "perhaps." Forty percent do not even believe that diet *might* be the most important factor. In other words, they're certain it's *not* the most important factor. One may conclude that their lack of nutritional education in medical school has made many of them close minded, 40 percent in fact. Fortunately, this attitude is changing. Many medical schools are now showing an interest in nutrition education. They are reconsidering the role of nutrition in medical education.

Congress is concerned about escalating health care expenditures and has recognized the need to intervene to improve public health and lower medical costs. The Pew Health Professions Commission has outlined the need for medical training to focus more on the population as a whole rather than be client-centered, as it is now. The commission also recommends that training be more interdisciplinary and *prevention oriented*.

So what does this mean for all of us? I'm not saying that you shouldn't listen to your doctor. That would be ridiculous. What I am saying is that we should know enough about nutrition and understand its effect on our health to work with our doctors in order to improve the health of our family. Knowledge is power, and the more we know, the more we can't choose NOT to know.

4

· · · · · · · · · · · ·

If You Build It,
They Will Come

It's better to have a little "whine" with your dinner for a few months than to give in to poor eating habits. And let's face it, Moms, we instilled those habits in the first place; we have a responsibility to undo them.—MARY BETH BORKOWSKI, NEW JERSEY

Teaching Your Child About Healthy Food

You may assume that you have little influence over your child's dietary choices, but recent studies done here in the United States and in Europe show that children, when given a choice, are much more likely to eat foods they eat regularly at home over the foods their best friends eat. The main conclusion was that the foods kids eat at home profoundly shape their dietary choices when they are away from home. Unfortunately, what most kids eat at home is not very healthy, either.

Most people know the difference between healthy food and junk food when they're shopping for themselves and their kids, but there are obstacles when it comes to putting healthy eating into practice. Does this sound familiar? You go shopping on Sunday armed with a very healthy shopping list focused on whole grains, fruits, and vegetables. As you fill up your shopping cart with all the well-intended healthy stuff for your kids, you add, for fun, devilish items like frozen pizza rolls, Pop-Tarts, and mesquite-flavored potato chips. You think, "We've gotta live it up once in a while, right? Besides, we'll be eating all of those grains, fruits, and vegetables to even it out." Well, that night, when you go to prepare your first meal with that fully stocked fridge of yours, you automatically reach for the fun pizza rolls. The next morning the kids grab the Pop-Tarts, and before you even get a chance to prepare lunch, Junior fills up on the mesquite-flavored potato chips. Your family's palates are now in party mode, and for the next few days, you guys can't even think about, much less eat, the formerly fresh spinach that is very close to its expiration date on the bottom shelf. When you finally run out of the junk food, the healthy stuff is now wilted. It's only Thursday, and you have to go shopping again. The result of this cycle is wasted food, wasted money, wasted time, and, worst of all, missed opportunity for your family to eat healthier.

Well, right off the bat, the first thing to do to break this cycle is not to buy the temptation foods. Try to exercise your strongest willpower when you're shopping. Keep the bad stuff out of sight, and it will automatically be out of mind. Don't think, "All right, I'll allow myself the pizza rolls if, and only if, I prepare and eat the brown rice and vegetables." Remember that our willpower is weakest when we're hungry. Don't challenge yourself to face moments like this. Shop like a mighty, unstoppable health warrior deflecting the onslaught of chips, dips, and lunch meats while you're on your way to the produce section. Besides, there are healthy versions of all of these forbidden foods. You just have to know where to find them.

Centered Food = Centered Behavior

Yin/yang, expansive/contractive, up/down, cold/hot, female/male—call it whatever you want. The ancient Chinese philosophy of yin/yang is connected to everything in the universe. The Chinese are perhaps best known for defining the world using this concept of duality, but an awareness of duality can be found in *every* culture and religion past and present. Yin and yang are used to symbolize and explain the law of change and unity of opposites in nature. Everything in the universe has two opposite aspects that are simultaneously in conflict and interdependent. People commonly think of yin and yang as opposing forces, but it is more appropriate to see them as a complementary pair. When we're cold, we crave warmth. When our lives become predictable, we crave surprise and passion. When we eat something salty (yang), we crave something sweet (yin). This is what your body does naturally to balance your life and the food you eat. It is one of the most basic laws of nature

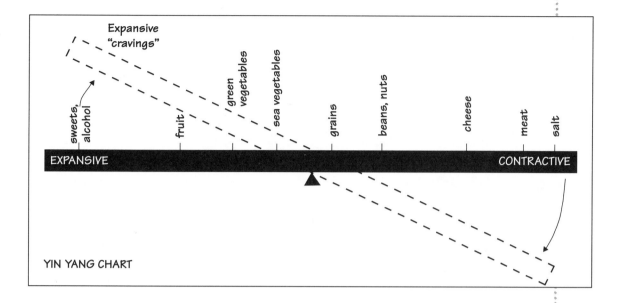

YIN YANG CHART

that for every action, there is an opposite and equal reaction. The more extreme an action, the more extreme the opposing action in order to find a balance. I definitely used to have extreme cravings in my diet. As soon as I satisfied one extreme, I automatically craved the other. When I was a kid, I constantly went back and forth between sugar and salt. Before I started eating the way I do now, after a very heavy meat meal (yang), the first thing I wanted was a sugary, puffy, creamy dessert (yin). Why do you think kids always want soda with their potato chips?

Problems arise when there is an imbalance between these two forces, whatever they may be. Many things can be attributed to disharmony in the forces of yin and yang, even divorce, bankruptcy, and, of course, disease. A healthy body depends on balance, and all diseases result from an imbalance of yin and yang, especially an imbalanced diet.

When I began studying food, I discovered that all food could be placed on a line divided by a center fulcrum, much like a seesaw. On one side of this imaginary seesaw are the expansive foods (yin) and on the other side are the contractive foods (yang). Foods on this seesaw can also be categorized in intensity—moderate (close to the center or fulcrum) or extreme (farther from the center). If you eat something moderate, you crave something from the other side that is also moderate. When you eat something extreme (like beef), you will crave something at the other end that is also extreme (like cola, chocolate, or beer). Extreme expansion balances extreme contraction, or sweet balances meat. This is the law of opposites. Balancing in the extremes is possible. It is, in fact, the way most people in America eat today. However, it consumes much more energy than eating and balancing foods closer to the center. Habitually eating from the extremes is wasteful, stressful, and exhausting. People can never understand why they have no energy to get through their day. They are worn out from swinging back and forth throughout their day between Starbucks and muffins in the morning, a ham and cheese sandwich for lunch, and a steak, baked potato, and dessert at dinner. Nor can parents understand why their children swing back and forth between being hyperactive and tired and cranky, both at home and at school. Could it be the constant seesaw between cereal, Happy Meals, pizza, cookies, candy, and fried chicken? No wonder so many of our kids are on Ritalin.

Extreme eating causes the body's blood quality to constantly fluctuate. The swing from yin to yang is too taxing. Our physical and psychological conditions become overstressed and weakened. Our body has a coping mechanism to handle these extremes. Over time, it naturally stores the excess (in order to minimize the shock to the body) in the form of fats and toxins, which eventually can crystallize to become cysts and tumors. This is why extreme foods (meat, cheese, butter, sugar, and alcohol) are connected to cancer, diabetes, and heart disease.

The best diet for you and your children is based on foods that are closest to the center. Notice that all the foods near the center are plant foods—whole grains, beans, vegetables, and fruit.

When we were kids, we were taught that a balanced diet was one with plenty of meat, eggs, whole milk, cheese, fresh green vegetables, and some fruit. As you can see, except for the fruit and vegetables, it's just the opposite. In fact, a "balanced" diet would put your body out of balance. It is a diet that is heavily weighted on the contractive (yang) end of the scale and leads to cravings for expansive (yin) foods like sugar, sweets, alcohol, and (in the extreme) drugs. Diets heavily weighted at one end affect behavior in specific ways. Extreme food leads to extreme behavior. Extreme and unbalanced diets tend to make you and your children more inclined to extreme feelings, extreme thoughts, and extreme actions. We all have the ability to control our behavior to some degree, but eating an extreme diet makes that self-control more difficult and leads to increased tension, stress, frustration, and eventually disease. Extreme foods also contribute to unnecessary violence. As people eat more and more extreme foods, their behavior becomes more intense and destructive. Of course, diet is not the only cause of violence or other extreme behavior, but an extreme diet can be a major contributor, especially when partnered with social problems at home or at school.

There is no question that extreme food such as meat, sugar, alcohol, and other drugs intensify the pent-up tension inside a person's body. Eating meat and sugar in the quantities found in the typical American diet leads to a noticeable increase in high blood pressure and heart disease, which affects 1 out of every 3 people.

Live Foods vs. Dead Foods

Dead food? What does that mean? Dead foods are foods that were once "live," "real" foods but have since been overprocessed to the point that they've lost their nutrition and vibrancy. As food is chopped, cooked, enriched, powdered, bleached, mixed (and whatever else food "manufacturers" do), it gets farther and farther from its natural state. It becomes, in fact, more and more *dead*. "Live" food, on the other hand, is food that came directly from the state that it was in while in nature. "Live" food is basically the same as whole food. Nearly everything in the produce section of the market is a live food, especially organic produce, because it contains no pesticides or other chemicals used to increase production and profits. Whole/live foods are not only in the produce section, though. Look at the ingredients on a container of good old-fashioned oatmeal. Its one and only ingredient is simply "oatmeal." That's another definition of a live/whole food; its only ingredient is itself. Our parents and grandparents ate nothing but live/whole foods. They were lucky because they had no choice. Processed foods hadn't become the norm yet. Our generation, and especially our children's generation, seem to be eating nothing but "dead" food. It's very expensive and less profitable to grow, ship, and market "live" food, so food producers sell us "dead" food.

The saddest part is that our culture has actually become accustomed to dead food, and most people's taste buds prefer it. But once you allow your taste buds to reacquaint themselves with food in its purest form, you'll start to have a renewed appreciation for live foods. They really do taste better. If we could transport our late great-grandparents in a time machine to sample today's standard American diet, they would barely recognize it as food. I know that trying to get your kids to learn to love "live," "real," "whole" food can be extremely difficult, but it's worth it. The farther away you get from eating natural grains and other whole foods, the worse it is for your health and your children's health.

For example, take something as common as a loaf of white bread. It's over-processed, overmilled, overpasteurized, and so far away from its live state that it's not going to add the same vibrancy to your health as something that's in its purer form. Sprouted whole grain bread is healthier than whole wheat, and whole wheat is more alive than white bread. The closer your bread is to a true complex carbo-hydrate (grains in their natural form), the better for your child's digestion and health.

The Hunza people of the Himalayas have always been a mystery to anthropol-ogists and nutritionists because they are stronger, healthier, and live longer than other people in the same region. Because their diet consists primarily of whole grains, vegetables, and fruits, and is nearly void of meat and refined sugar and flour, it was assumed diet was the reason for this. My *Total Health Makeover* book must be selling well at the Barnes and Noble in Kathmandu. (Actually, the Hunzas occasionally eat meat in very small quantities in winter—so they are close, but not true THMers.)

Based on this theory of a superior diet, an experiment was conducted several years ago using two groups of rats. One group ate a diet typical of the Hunzas, and the other group of rats was fed a diet like the rest of the native population, people living in other parts of India, and the British lower class, who typically ate refined carbohydrates.

As expected, the rats fed the Hunza diet were healthy, disease free, grew and mated normally, and had healthy offspring. The rats fed the refined food diets had all kinds of problems: pneumonia, anemia, sinusitis, ulcers, goiter, heart dis-ease, and premature birth. It was also observed during the experiment that the disposition of the Hunza rats was gentle, playful, and affectionate. They seemed to get along well with each other and were even affectionate with their handlers. This was not expected before the experiment. On the other hand, the other group, the junk food rats, were described as irritable and vicious. In fact, some even turned to cannibalism. (Yikes!) This was one of the earliest experiments of its kind.

The following have been associated with eating refined foods in the many experiments done since:

- ✦ Ulcer, tumors, and cancer of the large intestine
- ✦ Heart and vascular disease (including varicose veins)
- ✦ Gallstones, appendicitis, and hemorrhoids
- ✦ Diabetes and hypoglycemia
- ✦ Obesity
- ✦ Tooth and gum disease
- ✦ Psychotic behavior
- ✦ Anxiety
- ✦ Apathy
- ✦ Depression
- ✦ Violent and antisocial behavior

It was found that many of these conditions improve considerably when refined foods are eliminated from a person's diet. There are reasons for this. Whole foods are high in nutrition and fiber. When you eat whole, high fiber foods, there is a smooth and continuous passage of food through your intestines. This leads to a regular, continuous firing of the nonspecific nerve fibers into your arousal system and more effective neuronal conduction. I know that sounds pretty technical, but what it means is that your "living" body and "living" digestive system know precisely what to do with "live" food. The fiber (aka roughage or bulk) stimulates the wavelike contractions that move food through the intestine. In addition to this, the bulkiness of high fiber foods keeps the colon expanded, which produces softer stools and easier bowel movements. All of these factors lead to a healthier digestive system and aid the healing and prevention of some digestive disorders like irritable bowel syndrome (IBD), hemorrhoids, and diverticulosis.

In contrast, when you eat a refined or a low fiber diet (lots of white flour, dairy, sugar, and meat), your digestive system gets confused. Movement in the intestines becomes interrupted and irregular. And the nerve fibers connected to the digestion arousal system becomes less reliable and less effective. In short, your digestive system doesn't work quite right. Over time, animal foods putrefy in the intestines and produce toxic by-products, which, if not quickly eliminated, cause biochemical and even behavioral disorders. Eventually, toxins build up during a lifetime and potentially lead to disease and death.

My children and I eat fruits and vegetables and whole grains every day. I always think of these live foods as something that gives you life. Dead food, in contrast, makes you tired. Your digestive system expends a great deal of energy to do its job. When it's functioning properly and breaking down the live food it was designed to do, it actually energizes you. When your digestive system is confused, it works overtime and drains all of your body's precious energy. After a typical American lunch, your child will be dead tired and irritable at school the rest of the day. That's why it is so important to feed your children as much live food as you possibly can.

If you eat a dead food diet of fast food, processed food, and junk food, it's not only highly processed, it's also full of fat and chemicals. The addition of chemicals is necessary to put back the flavor that was processed out. Take your typical fast food burger. Each layer has some processing done to it (even the pickle). The grain in the white bun has been milled down. The French fries are coated in oil. The hamburger is long dead. Now I'm not saying that you and your kids should eat only raw foods all the time, and all their vegetables should be eaten raw. That's boring. I'm just asking you to become more aware of the kinds of foods you're consuming. For the next week or so, keep track of all foods you and your family eat. Make a list with two columns. One column for all the whole foods and the other for processed foods. Get ready. This can be a real eye-opener for some people.

The Difference Between Sustenance Foods and Pleasure Foods

All foods should be a pleasure to eat, but there are certain foods that can be classified as "pleasure foods." Pleasure foods are all those foods that are not the main foods of your diet that sustain life, but rather the extra filler foods that give you emotional satisfaction because they taste good, they're social, or they're part of our culture. You know these foods: cookies, candy, guacamole and chips, snack foods. (Yes, they're very much a part of my family's life, too.) Pleasure foods have to be part of any eating lifestyle. The real problem is that for some people it is their only eating lifestyle.

The idea is to put an end to that mindless eating that many families do in front of the television set, where it's just gut fill. At the end of the evening, all that is left are those empty bags of potato chips or containers of ice cream. No question about it, we've all been there. Fun little pleasure foods should still be part of your family's health, but you are going to have to be more conscious of them.

Whole Foods

Over the years, people have often said to me things like "If you don't eat meat, dairy, sugar, or any processed foods, what's left?" People are under the impression that eating the way I do requires discipline and an adjustment to a severely limited choice of foods. What they don't realize is that after you have freed yourself from those deadly American staples (the Health Robbers, as I like to call them), you begin to discover what seems to be an unlimited variety of foods you have either forgotten about or never knew existed. It turns out that my diet seemed most limited when I was eating a typical American diet in my teens and early twenties.

Fruits and Vegetables

There is so much advice out there about what we should and shouldn't eat. And you can find experts on both sides of just about every dietary issue in the world. Some nutritionists recommend a high carbohydrate diet; others emphasize a high protein diet. Some say it's necessary for us to take dietary supplements; others say it's a waste of time. And no matter what the issue is, there's always at least *some* evidence supporting both sides. This is the case with every dietary issue— except one. *Everybody* agrees that eating a diet rich in fruits and vegetables is an essential part of every healthy eating plan. Think about it. It would be very difficult to find anyone who disagrees with that statement. And it's not even the fact that fruits and vegetables supply the vitamins, minerals, phytochemicals, and fiber that are essential to human growth and vitality. Or that a high consumption of fruits and vegetables have been found by the U.S. Department of Health and Human Services, the U.S. Department of Agriculture, and the National Academy of Sciences to lower your risk for cancer and heart disease (and probably every other major disease). These are all just some of the many benefits that come from the fact that fruits and vegetables are the food that we humans are designed to eat— period.

Fruits and vegetable are loaded with phytochemicals. As early as 1980, the

National Cancer Institute Chemoprevention Program of the Division of Cancer Prevention and Control began evaluating phytochemicals and their properties for preventing and treating diseases. Researchers have long known that there are phytochemicals present in plants for their protection but only recently have they been recommended as protection against human disease. What exactly are phytochemicals? Phytochemicals are a natural bioactive compound found in plant foods that contain protective, disease-preventing compounds. Although phytochemicals are not classified as nutrients, they are known to contain properties that aid in disease prevention. Research suggests that phytochemicals may help slow the aging process and reduce the risk of many diseases, including cancer, heart disease, stroke, high blood pressure, cataracts, osteoporosis, and urinary tract infections. More than 900 different phytochemicals have been identified in food. It is estimated that there may be more than 100 different phytochemicals in just one serving of vegetables.

Phyto is a Greek word that means "plant"; therefore, phytochemical literally means plant-chemical. Don't let the word "chemical" fool you. These are not like artificial additives or other chemicals that are added to food; they're naturally occurring chemicals found in foods like fruits, vegetables, and grains. The brightest colored fruits and vegetables often contain the most phytochemicals.

Phytochemicals are often consumed in supplements; however, consumption of supplements containing phytochemicals will only provide minimal components in an unnatural, concentrated form—not the diversity of compounds that occur naturally in whole fruits and vegetables. Phytochemicals complement, aid, and stimulate the immune system, the detoxification of enzymes, and hormone metabolism, and have an antioxidant, antibacterial, and antiviral effect.

Micronutrients are vitamins and minerals that have been found to greatly benefit overall health, mental attitude, and even longevity. Flavonoids and carotenoids are the two largest categories of micronutrients. There are twelve categories of flavonoids that total over 20,000 micronutrients. One plant alone may contain over a hundred types of flavenoids. There are five categories of carotenoids, totaling over 600 micronutrients. Carotenoids are especially helpful in fighting cancer, heart disease, and other degenerative diseases.

The National Cancer Institute, a branch of the National Institutes of Health, recommends eating at least five servings of fruits and vegetables a day. Similarly, the U.S. Department of Agriculture recommends five to nine servings a day. Okay, since we're all pretty much in agreement here, let's get down to business and stock your kitchen with an abundance of F's and V's, and more important, make a plan for you and your kids to eat them consistently.

The first choice for fruits and vegetables should be whatever is grown somewhat locally, is in season, and organic, if possible. Think of these three as priorities, not rules. The best way to find out what's local, in season, or organic is to carefully read the signs and ask the produce manager at your local Whole Foods Market, Wild Oats, or other produce market or supermarket that's comparable. Generally, it's best to select fruits and vegetables that are evenly colored, vibrant, and unblemished. The problem here is that conventional produce would usually win a beauty contest against the organic produce. Since you're not taking it to the senior prom, choose the organic produce anyway, but choose the best-looking among them. Conventional produce usually looks better than organic because industrial farmers and packers have tampered with nature in the form of chemicals, pesticides, and/or waxes for appearance and preservation.

> Today nearly three-fourths of grocery stores and supermarkets sell organic and natural foods, according to research done by the Food Marketing Institute in 1999.
>
> *Natural Health*, March 2001

Beans and Legumes

Beans and legumes are a popular staple throughout the world because they're abundant, inexpensive, and a wonderful source of protein and soluble fiber. Since the seventies, the health benefits of dietary fiber have become increasingly apparent. Beans and legumes are loaded with protein like animal meats, but unlike meat, they are not loaded with fat and calories. Beans and legumes can really add flavor and nutrition to your cooking, and best of all, kids love them! In fact, I sent edamame (boiled soybeans) to school for my son's healthy snack, and I had mothers calling me asking, "What did the kids eat today that looked like green M&Ms? They loved them!"

Beans and legumes are an excellent source of soluble fiber, the same sticky fiber found in oat products that helps direct insulin into individual cells and out of the bloodstream. (Highest in fiber are black-eyed peas, kidney beans, chickpeas, lima beans, and black beans.) Beans/legumes lower cholesterol, maintain stable blood sugar levels, and may help prevent cancer, heart disease, diabetes mellitus, gastrointestinal disease, obesity, and hypertension. They also contain several anticancer compounds: lignins, saponins, isoflavones, phytic acid, and protease

PHYTOCHEMICALS IN FRUITS AND VEGETABLES

Carotenoids in Fruits and Vegetables

Carotenoid	Benefit	Found In
Beta-carotene	Helps to slow aging process, reduces risk of certain types of cancer, improves lung function, reduces complications associated with diabetes.	Mango, cantaloupe, apricots, papaya, kiwifruit, carrots, pumpkins, sweet potatoes, winter squash, broccoli, spinach, kale.
Lutein	Maintains vision as we age, reduces risk of cataracts, reduces risk of certain types of cancer.	Kale, spinach, collard greens, kiwifruit, broccoli, brussels sprouts, Swiss chard, romaine lettuce.
Lycopene	Reduces risk of prostate cancer and heart disease.	Tomatoes, red peppers, watermelon, grapefruit.
Zeaxanthin	Helps prevent macular degeneration (the leading cause of visual impairment in people over 50); prevents certain types of cancer.	Corn, spinach, winter squash, egg yolks.

Flavonoids in Fruits and Vegetables

Flavonoid	Benefit	Found In
Anthocyanin	Protects against signs of aging, helps prevent urinary tract infections.	Blueberries, cranberries, cherries, strawberries, kiwifruit, plums.
Hesperidin	Protects against heart disease.	Oranges, grapefruit, tangerines, lemons, limes, mandarins, tangelos.
Resveratrol	Reduces risk of heart disease, cancer, blood clots, and stroke.	Red grapes.
Quercetin	Reduces inflammation associated with allergies, inhibits the growth of head and neck cancers, protects lungs from pollutants and cigarette smoke.	Apples, pears, cherries, grapes, onions, kale, broccoli, leaf lettuce, garlic, green tea, red wine.
Tangeritin	Prevents cancers of the head and neck.	Citrus fruits.

PHYTOCHEMICALS IN FRUITS AND VEGETABLES

Flavonoid	Benefit	Found In
Phenolic compounds	May reduce the risk of heart disease and certain types of cancer.	Berries, prunes, red grapes, kiwifruit, currants, apples, tomatoes.
Ellagic acid	May reduce the risk of certain types of cancer, decrease cholesterol levels.	Red grapes, kiwifruit, blueberries, raspberries, strawberries, blackberries, currants.
Sulphoraphane	May reduce the risk of colon cancer.	Broccoli, cauliflower, kale, brussels sprouts, cabbage, bok choy, collard greens, turnips.
Limonene	Protects lungs and reduces the risk of certain types of cancer.	In rinds and edible white membranes of oranges, grapefruit, tangerines, lemons, limes.
Indoles	May reduce the risk of certain types of cancer, including breast cancer.	Broccoli, cauliflower, kale, brussels sprouts, cabbage, bok choy, collard greens, watercress, turnips.
Allium Compounds	May reduce the risk of certain types of cancer, lower cholesterol and blood pressure.	Garlic, onions, chives, leeks, scallions.

inhibitors. Protease inhibitors hinder cancer cells in their early stages and isoflavones help neutralize the powerful estrogens that can lead to breast cancer.

Beans were once called the "poor man's meat." (I think that's so funny. Meat really should be called the "unhealthy man's beans.") Legumes and beans don't really have that reputation anymore because of our awareness of their many benefits and cooking versatility. But it's not enough. Most Americans only consume half the recommended twenty to thirty-five grams of fiber by the United States Department of Agriculture (USDA). An increase in bean consumption alone would change that trend.

Beans are similar in nutritional and calorie content (about ninety-five calories per cooked half cup) yet are different in taste. You can experiment to find your family's favorite beans or legumes and not have to worry much about whether it's more or less nutritional than another bean. Beans have no cholesterol, are almost totally free of fat, and are a dense source of plant protein. (What's not to love!) Beans/legumes contain substantial amounts of calcium, iron, potassium, phosphorus, zinc, magnesium, and B vitamins. A single cup of lentils contains 25 percent of the RDA (recommended daily allowance) of iron for a woman.

Beans are also great for weight management. A meal made primarily with beans keeps insulin levels low. A rise in insulin triggers hunger. Beans keep appetites in check because they tend to keep insulin in check. Beans can also keep diabetes under control. Diabetes mellitus is characterized by elevated blood sugar. The soluble fiber in beans tends to coagulate the food in the intestines, which slows the passage of glucose from food into the cells and results in a slow rise in blood sugar. Thanks to an increase in beans and soluble fiber, some individuals with diabetes mellitus have been able to reduce or discontinue their hypoglycemic medications since less insulin is needed to control blood sugar.

The fiber found in beans decreases the risk of our number one killers, heart disease and stroke, because it lowers blood fats, bad cholesterol, and blood pressure; improves blood sugar; and helps prevent obesity. Research conducted at the University of Kentucky concluded that one cup of beans daily lowers serum cholesterol about 10 percent after twenty-one days.

Okay, so is there anything wrong with beans and legumes? Well, no . . . not exactly! There is a certain prejudice against them thanks to comedians like Mel Brooks and his famous scene from *Blazing Saddles*. But this is not really fair. Flatulence and gastrointestinal discomfort can be associated with eating beans because some people may lack the enzymes needed to digest certain complex bean sugars known as oligosaccharides. When these undigested sugars reach the intestine, they are broken down by bacteria, which produce carbon dioxide, hydrogen, and other gases. The problem often comes not from the beans or legumes themselves, but from bad dietary combinations consumed with the beans. Other causes are overeating and having a digestive system that is unfamiliar with beans. So, before you turn away from beans because you fear your friends and loved ones will turn away from you, try the following:

◆ Keep meals light. Your digestive system can't function properly when it is overloaded.

✦ Don't mix beans with too many foods that don't combine well with them—especially fruits, sweets, and dairy products (I'm trying to get you to reconsider those, anyway).

✦ If you don't eat beans frequently, give your body time to adjust by eating a little at first, and gradually increase the amount you consume. Your body can build up the enzymes required to digest beans over time.

Right now genetic engineers are working on new varieties of "gasless beans." Leave it to scientists and food producers to take a perfect food in nature and find a way to change its molecular structure in search of production and profit. Haven't they learned? It's the trans fatty acid story all over again. Eventually, I'm sure they'll find a bean that will remove gas, but replace it with a nice big tumor.

Whole Grains

When you think of foods in the whole grain category, what's the first thing you think of? Most Americans think of breads, pastas, cereals, and rice. These are the four foods typically pictured in the government's food pyramid chart in the grain section. It's the largest and most highly recommended section (for quantity and frequency of consumption) by nearly every nutrition expert. Most parents are confident that their children are "eating their grains," because American kids actually do consume a great deal of bread, cereals, pastas, muffins, etc. Unfortunately, as I stated earlier, only 2 percent of the flour consumed in this country is whole grain. The other 98 percent is processed. "Real" whole grains are actually pretty foreign to most Americans.

This is a problem because refining (see page 34 for further explanation) removes the bran and germ, leaving only the inside core, the endosperm. Without all three, digestion becomes less efficient and the most beneficial elements (protein, complex carbohydrates, unsaturated fats, B-complex vitamins, vitamin E, and iron) become waste products at the refining plant along with all that wonderful intestine-scrubbing fiber. It's very sad.

On the average, twenty-four ingredients are removed during refining. So the essential enzymes, nutrients, and fiber we assume our children are getting from their "grains" have been depleted during processing and refining.

Not all products are refined equally; some are more refined than others. Keep in mind that the more of the kernel that is left intact, the more natural heart-healthy

BEANS AND LEGUMES PREPARATION TIPS

An important part of dried bean preparation is the preliminary soaking. Every bean with the exception of split peas and lentils should be soaked thoroughly before cooking. It is optimal to soak them overnight, but if it's not possible, try to soak larger, denser beans for 8 hours or more and smaller beans for at least 4 hours.

After picking through the dried beans and removing any withered ones, cover them with cold water and remove any beans that float to the top. Rinse as many times as needed to leave the water clear.

Note: Cooking times vary. The following are suggestions. You should really cook until beans are tender or to your liking. The water amounts are suggestions as well. The water will be discarded after the beans are cooked, so it's not essential to have measurements exact.

Bean	Description	Cooking Instructions
Adzuki	Small, oval, dark red beans. They have a nutlike flavor and light texture. Easily digestible.	Cook 1 cup dried beans in 4 quarts water for 1 hour and 15 minutes. Yields 2 cups.
Black	Medium-size oval beans. Soft texture. Great in soups.	Cook 1 cup dried beans in 3 quarts water for 1½ hours. Yields 2 cups.
Black-eyed peas	Small white bean with one black spot (the eye). A mealy texture. Great in stuffings and soups.	Cook 1 cup dried beans in 2¼ quarts water for 1 hour. Yields 2 cups.
Cannellini	Just like a white kidney bean. A nutty flavor. Prominently used in many Italian dishes.	Cook 1 cup dried beans in 1 quart water for 1½ to 2 hours. Yields 2 cups.
Fava (Broad)	Lightish brown in color, flat and kidney-shaped. Wonderful pureed. Remove the skins after cooking.	Cook 1 cup dried beans in 4 quarts water for 1½ hours. Yields 2 cups.
Garbanzo (Chickpeas)	Tan and round. They have a really hearty flavor. Used to make hummus and enhance the flavor of soups and salads.	Cook 1 cup dried beans in 4 quarts water for 2 to 3 hours. Yields 2 cups.
Kidney	Red bean with a kidney shape. Used in chili, salads, soups, and stews.	Cook 1 cup dried beans in 2 quarts water for 2 hours. Yields 2 cups.
Lentils	Many varieties. Shaped like tiny disks. The most common are red, brown, and green. Commonly used in Middle Eastern dishes.	Cook 1 cup dried beans in 4 cups water for 1 hour. Yields 2¾ cups.

BEANS AND LEGUMES PREPARATIONS TIPS		
Bean	**Description**	**Cooking Instructions**
Lima	Light green in color and flat. They come large and small and have a starchy texture.	Cook 1 cup dried beans in 2 quarts water for 1½ hours. Yields 2¾ cups.
Navy	Small and white. Very versatile. Slightly granular texture.	Cook 1 cup dried beans in 3½ quarts water for 1½ to 2 hours. Yields 2 cups.
Pinto	Large oval bean with a brown skin. Earthy flavor. Commonly in Spanish, Mexican, and southwestern dishes.	Cook 1 cup dried beans in 2 quarts water for 1½ to 2 hours. Yields 2 cups.
Red	Dark red and medium-size ovals. Similar to kidney beans. Used in many Mexican dishes.	Cook 1 cup dried beans in 2 quarts water for 1½ to 2 hours. Yields 2 cups.
Soybeans	Light green oval-like beans that come in a pea pod. One of the earth's most nutritious foods. Used to make tofu and miso.	Cook 1 cup dried beans in 3½ quarts water for 3 to 4 hours. Yields 2 cups.
Split peas	Small beans that come in yellow and green. Can be split or used whole. Great in soups.	Cook 1 cup dried beans in 4 cups water for 40 to 50 minutes. Yields 2 cups.
White (Great Northern)	Large and white with a grainy texture. Good in stews and hearty dishes.	Cook 1 cup dried beans in 3½ quarts water for 1 hour and 15 minutes. Yields 2 cups.

fiber, nutrition, and enzymes are left for your children's bodies. It can be very challenging when striving to limit most of your family's grain consumption to fit in the 2 percent "whole grains only" category and not the 98 percent "refined junk" category.

It's challenging, but you certainly can do it. And boy, is it worth it when you do. You'll quickly notice a visible improvement in your family's energy, sleep habits, bowel regularity, and overall health and temperament. This doesn't mean that you can't continue to serve breads, pastas, rice, and cereals. It just means you have to be more selective at the market to find more unrefined products, and be a little more creative in the kitchen. If you want to be certain you're getting whole

GRAINS PRIMER

Grain	Description	Cooking Instructions
Amaranth	An Aztec grain with a sticky texture. Great in combination with other grains.	Cook 1 cup amaranth in 2½ cups water for 20 minutes. Yields 3 cups.
Barley	Beige kernels with extremely mild flavor and soft texture. Great as a side dish or added to soup.	Cook 1 cup barley in 2 cups water for 15 minutes. Yields 3 cups.
Buckwheat	Whole kernels with an earthy flavor. Roasted buckwheat is kasha and makes a great pilaf.	Cook 1 cup buckwheat in 2 cups water for 15 minutes. Yields 2½ cups.
Cornmeal	White or yellow corn kernels ground to a grainy powder. Sweet. Great in breads.	Cook 1 cup cornmeal in 4 cups water for 30 minutes. Yields 4 cups.
Millet	Small, light brown, whole kernels. Chewy and served like rice.	Cook 1 cup millet in 4 cups water for 30 minutes. Yields 4 cups.
Oats	Whole oat grain; nutty flavor and chewy texture. Wonderful breakfast food. Major claims of lowering cholesterol.	Cook 1 cup oats in 4 cups water for 60 minutes. Yields 4 cups.
Quinoa	Light yellow seed about the size of rice. Sweet flavor and soft texture. A whole protein in itself. Great as a salad base.	Cook 1 cup quinoa in 2 cups water for 15 minutes. Yields 3 cups.
Rice (brown)	Dark rice that is sweet and has hints of nut. Always a wonderful side dish.	Cook 1 cup brown rice in 2 cups water for 60 minutes. Yields 3 cups.
Rye berries	Small brown seedlike berries. A chewy grain that sucks the fat right out of your body (in my opinion). This is used in the rice and rye staple.	Cook 1 cup rye berries in 2½ cups water for 25 minutes. Yields 3 cups.
Wheat berries	Unprocessed whole-wheat kernels. Slightly chewy and great for baking.	Cook 1 cup wheat berries in 3 cups water for 2 hours. Yields 3 cups.
Wild rice	Long dark or light kernels with an earthy flavor.	Cook 1 cup wild rice in 2½ cups water for 50 minutes. Yields 3 cups.

grains, simply buy all your grains in the raw and cook and prepare them yourself. As you're planning meals for your family, you should think of grains as the centerpiece of most meals. It is after all the most important food group. For most grains, the basic recipe for preparation is approximately 2 parts water to 1 part grain. Bring the water to a boil, add the grain, cover, and simmer on low heat, until the water is absorbed (approximately 15 to 30 minutes depending on the grain). The more often you cook it, the better you will be able to judge how long it will take on your stove. When the grain is done, remove it from the heat, uncover the pot, and allow it to cool without stirring. The best way to cook grains is to get a rice cooker. It's so simple to use, and you'll make perfect rice every time. They are widely available at many department stores, appliance stores, and even drugstores.

Everybody's familiar with wheat, rice, and even oats; but what about amaranth, barley, buckwheat, quinoa, or rye? At one time or another, you should try all of these. You never know. You may find a wonderful new taste sensation. Opposite is a little grain-by-grain breakdown to get you familiar with the world of whole grains.

Lean Proteins

I firmly believe that your children can get all the protein they will ever need exclusively from plant sources: beans, legumes, nuts, grains, and from some fruits and vegetables. However, eating a totally vegan diet (no animal products whatsoever including fish) is a little strict for most people. I myself eat some kinds of fish (but rarely shellfish). It is the only animal protein I eat. I have not had dairy, beef, pork, veal, turkey, chicken, or any other fowl in over twenty years. I do allow my sons to eat fish and occasionally a little free-range organic chicken and turkey. In this section I would like to discuss which animal proteins I believe are good (or at least acceptable) for eating.

To begin with, I advise against *any* consumption of *any* products associated with cows, pigs, and sheep—period. All the reasons I mentioned in Chapter 2, plus all the horror stories about mad-cow disease and the foot-and-mouth plague we have been reading about in the news lately, should be enough to turn you off to eating those animals.

That pretty much leaves us with poultry and fish. I recommend turkey and chicken for kids only if it is free-range and organic. I know that sounds a little strict, but in all honesty, it would be healthier for you and your family than the alternative—steroid and antibiotic injected commercial (nonorganic) supermarket or fast food chicken or turkey without trimming all the skin, grease, and fat. With these, you are getting comparable amounts of saturated fats, cholesterol, hormones, and chemicals.

Finally, let's talk about fish. It is a wonderful protein source, much lower in saturated fats than beef, pork, or chicken and less concentrated and much easier to digest. Many fish contain the kind of fat (omega-3 essential fatty acids) that is even good for your health. These fats appear to protect against heart disease, cancer, arthritis, and even mental disorders. They are found in salmon, sardines, herring, and mackerel.

In a perfect world, it would be fine, even great, to give generous amounts and a wide variety of fish to your kids. But this is certainly not a perfect world, and there are many things to worry about when considering fish consumption: contaminants, toxins, mercury content, oil spills, and fishing and fish farming methods. Before getting overly paranoid about all this, keep in mind that some fish are better than others, and there is a lot of controversy about which fish are dangerous and which are safe. For the most part, eat all fish in moderation, and you will reduce the risk of toxic buildup. The biggest concern of all is methyl mercury. Bacteria in the water convert inorganic mercury into toxic methyl mercury. Methyl mercury toxicity levels increase each time a larger fish eats a smaller one, so the higher a fish is on the food chain, the higher the toxicity risk. Ocean fish seem to be safer than fish from lakes, rivers, and streams because the ocean has less pollution. Farm-raised fish at one time were the safest choice, but many profit-minded fish farmers are using techniques (such as fertility drugs and antibiotics) these days that are not so different from chicken and beef producers. Shellfish are risky because they are bottom feeders and contain much of the pollutants, bacteria, and even some viruses like hepatitis, meningitis, and typhoid. In general, my advice is to stay away from shellfish. Don't eat fish every day, and when you do, lean toward ocean fish (smaller variety preferred), freshwater fish that you know come from safe waters, and organically raised farm fish. How do you find out which is which? Ask the manager in the fish department in your supermarket. Don't be afraid. They may really enjoy getting a chance to show off some of their knowledge.

When it comes to actually selecting fish at the market, there are several things to keep in mind. Freshness is very important. Start by asking the manager what the "catch of the day" is. If you are planning ahead, you can also ask about the store's delivery schedule for any specific fish. There is nothing wrong with asking questions. Every day counts with seafood. If you've ever tasted fish immediately after it came from the sea, you know exactly what I mean. Ask if any fish contain chemicals or preservatives. Some markets do this to increase shelf life, but it's not worth it. Without any preservatives, fish will last a maximum of 3 days. So buy it and make sure you eat it within that time frame (or else freeze it immediately). Don't settle for additives if you don't have to.

When selecting fresh fish, don't select anything that has a strong or unpleasant odor. Fish will have a distinctive smell if it's old. It will also be discolored yellow, brown, or black. Avoid fish with a filmy texture, too. Fish should have a fresh, clean feel to it. If it feels slimy to the touch, this means it has been sitting a while, and it's a little tired now. Fish that has gone bad will have an iodine smell and/or taste. If you happen to buy some bad fish, let your market know. They should be happy to refund your money. Most important, trust your instincts, eyes, fingers, and nose.

"Legal" Sugars

Kids love their sweets. What do children think about while they are having dinner? What they're going to have for dessert! What are most desserts made of? SUGAR! We already know how bad refined white sugar is. It has been blamed for hyperactivity, diabetes, hypoglycemia, severe mood swings, decreased brain function, serious digestion problems, yeast infections, obesity, and tooth decay. It depletes your body of all the B vitamins. It leaches calcium from your hair, bones, blood, and teeth, interferes with the absorption of calcium, protein, and other important minerals in the body, and retards the growth of valuable intestinal bacteria. And finally, sugar has a fermenting effect in your stomach. It stops the secretion of gastric juices and inhibits the mouth's ability to digest.

Okay! You've got a great kid who is pure joy to be with and she craves luscious candies and desserts that you really want to give her, but you know you can't. What's a parent to do? Sugar substitutes perhaps? There are many types of sugar substitutes out there, but you have to be careful because many are basically the same thing or almost as bad as refined white sugar. Some of these to watch out

SWEETENER CONVERSION CHART

Sweetener	Source/Taste	Form	Relative Sweetness
White sugar	Pure sweetness. Highly refined from sugar cane.	Granulated	1
Brown sugar	White sugar with a dye job. Slight molasses taste.	Granulated	1
Fructose	From corn. Very sweet.	Granulated	2
Honey	Extracted from flower nectar by bees. It's 20 to 60 percent sweeter than sugar, so use less.	Honeycomb, thick liquid, or cream	1.3
Maple syrup	Drawn from the sap of maple trees. Use only pure U.S. organic syrup to avoid formaldehyde and additives.	Syrup	0.6
Maple sugar	Dehydrated maple syrup.	Granulated	0.6
Barley malt	Sprouted barley. Strong distinctive flavor (like molasses).	Dark liquid	0.6
Brown rice syrup	Brown rice and various enzymes. Mild butterscotch flavor.	Thick liquid	0.7
Fruit juice concentrate	Peach, pear, grape, pineapple are most common.	Syrup or liquid	1.3
Molasses	Light and Barbados have lighter molasses taste than sorghum or blackstrap.	Syrup	0.6

Substitution for 1 Cup Sugar	Reduction of Total Liquid	Additional Comments
		May not be vegetarian. Beef bone used in some refineries. (Not recommended.)
		Same as white sugar. (Not recommended.)
		Highly refined. Sweetness unstable. (Not recommended.)
⅔ to ¾ cup	⅛ to ¼ cup. Add ¼ teaspoon of baking soda per cup honey.	Reduce oven 25 degrees and adjust the baking time.
¾ to 1 cup	⅛ to ¼ cup. Add ¼ teaspoon of baking soda per cup maple syrup.	Use in all baked goods. The moisture retention makes it especially good in cakes.
1 cup	No reduction of liquid. Add ⅛ teaspoon of baking soda per cup maple sugar.	Use in all baked goods. Store in airtight container and sift before using.
1⅓ to 1½ cups	¼ cup. Add ¼ teaspoon of baking soda per cup barley malt.	Stay away from barley/corn malt syrup. Buy only 100 percent barley malt. Organic available.
1⅓ to 1½ cups	¼ cup per cup brown rice syrup. ¼ teaspoon of baking soda per cup brown rice syrup.	Baked goods with brown rice syrup tend to be hard or very crisp. Combine with another sweetener such as maple for cakes.
⅔ cup	⅓ cup per cup of fruit sweetener. Add ¼ teaspoon of baking soda per cup fruit juice concentrate.	Reduce oven 25 degrees. Store in refrigerator but use at room temperature.
½ cup		Good in corn muffins, rye bread, gingerbread, and cookies

	SWEETENER CONVERSION CHART *(continued)*		
Sweetener	Source/Taste	Form	Relative Sweetness
Date sugar	Ground, dehydrated dates.	Granulated	0.6
Sucanat or Rapadura	Organic evaporated cane juice. Minerals and molasses are retained.	Granulated	1
Stevia	A perennial shrub of the aster family.	Whole or broken leaves, coarse ground, powder extract, or liquid extract	8 to 300 times, depending on quality and whether it is leaf or extract

for are corn syrup, brown sugar (that's just white sugar with a dye job), glucose, sucrose, and dextrose. Also, make sure you stay away from chemical sweeteners like saccharine, aspartame, and Acesulfame K. All three have been linked to cancer, and some are linked to memory loss and impaired brain function. Okay, now what?

Well, welcome to the wonderful world of healthier sugar substitutes! There are some terrific natural sweeteners that contain nutrients and minerals that sugar lost a long time ago at the refinery. They metabolize much slower in your child's body so she won't have that sugar rush–sugar crash syndrome like she does on refined sugar or as I like to call it, "kiddie cocaine."

Natural sweeteners include raw, unfiltered honey; maple syrup; maple sugar; Sucanat; barley malt; rice syrup; stevia; and agave. Some are more refined than others, making them a less desirable choice for your kids.

One final word of caution on sweets for your kids: don't think of these sugar substitutes as health food. They should still be treated a bit like a devilish treat, but they are definitely a big improvement over refined white sugar. If you really want to satisfy your kids' sweet tooth and not feel guilty about it, stock your refrigerator with an assortment of their favorite fruits. In addition, keep a bowl of fruit in plain sight at all times so they'll reach for one whenever they get the urge. Try a few dried fruits in moderation, too. And try putting some fruits in the

Substitution for 1 Cup Sugar	Reduction of Total Liquid	Additional Comments
1 cup		Add hot water to dissolve date sugars before using. Use in crisps, crunches, as sprinkle or topping. Purchase date sugar made from unsulfured, organically grown dates.
1 cup		Sift prior to using.
1 teaspoon	Experiment in converting recipes, adjusting liquid and dry ingredients to make up for lack of bulk.	May soon be in easier form to use. Significantly enhances the flavor and nutritional value of food.

freezer (like grapes, cherries, or bananas). Kids love frozen fruits, especially on a hot summer day.

Refer to the chart on pages 86–89 to help you sort out many of the most popular natural sweeteners.

Healthy Fats

As I stated earlier in Chapter 2, fat is a necessary part of a healthy diet. In fact, it's as necessary as protein and carbohydrates for our bodies to function properly, and it provides the most concentrated source of energy. Don't get me wrong here. I'm not recommending you fill the cookie jar with macadamia nuts or cashews. Children do need fat—but probably not as much as they typically eat. I recommend about 25 to 30 percent of their diet, depending on their BMI (Body Mass Index—a measurement of weight in relation to a person's height and age. See Chapter 1). Okay, we know kids need fat, so let's talk about the best (and worst) ways for them to get it.

Just as there are good and bad proteins, good and bad carbohydrates, and good and bad sweets, there are most definitely good and bad fats. It would probably be more appropriate to say there are good, bad, and *really* bad fats. The bad fats (not recommended) would be the saturated fats, which are found primarily in animal fats in meats, poultry, dairy, eggs, and butter. In this category the only fats from plant sources are saturated fats found in palm and coconut oil. They are not recommended even though they are plant based. Saturated fats raise LDL ("bad") cholesterol and clog arteries, leading to heart disease and stroke. They may also increase the risk of colon and prostate cancers.

Even though saturated fats are bad, there is a category of fats that is probably worse, the really bad fats—trans fatty acids. Earlier in this century, scientists found a way to make unsaturated fats behave like saturated fats by bombarding the unsaturated fat molecules with hydrogen. This is the process of hydrogenation. It increases the stability of a fat or oil, which is important in cooking and extending a product's shelf life. (For more on this process, see page 48.) There is really nothing beneficial for us in trans fat; this process only benefits the food producers. What they do for us is raise our bad cholesterol, lower our good cholesterol (HDL), harden our arteries over time, and they have probably contributed a great deal to the rampant growth of heart disease in our society in the last half of this century. Trans fats have been linked to several cancers, including colon and breast cancer. Keeping your family away from trans fats in not impossible. Shop in health food stores and carefully read the labels. Earth Balance, the "butter substitute" I have been recommending lately, does not contain hydrogenated oils.

You know about the bad fats and the *really* bad fats to keep far away from your kids. Let's get to the ones they *should* have in moderation, the good fats, aka the unsaturated fats. These fats actually lower the LDL ("bad") cholesterol. Mono-unsaturated fat is found in the following: olive oil, cashews, macadamias, almonds, and avocados. Omega-3 essential fatty acids are found in salmon, sardines, herring, mackerel, and walnuts. (For more information on fat, refer to Chapter 2.) Use the chart opposite as your guide to oils.

Encouraging Five Fruits and Vegetables Before Pleasure Foods

Last year I had the wonderful opportunity to speak in front of a large group of people in San Diego for the Healthy Dining Organization. This is an organization that has been given a grant by the government to encourage restaurants to create

IDEAL USES FOR NATURAL OILS

Oil	Taste and Properties	Culinary Uses
Almond	Strong, toasted nut; low smoke point	Excellent in salad dressings or chicken salad, drizzled over fish, or in nut-flavored baked goods; not suitable for deep-frying
Avocado	Rich, warm; high smoke point	Excellent in salads, on pasta; suitable for fast-frying, sautéing, and deep-frying
Canola	Light, clear, bland; high smoke point; all-purpose	Blends well for mayonnaise and dressings; especially good for baking
Corn	Pleasant "corny" flavor; general use	Good for baking (especially piecrusts), cooking, and making popcorn
Olive	Distinctive, fruity; all-purpose	Good for frying, sautéing, salad dressings, pasta sauces, some baking; not suitable for deep-frying
Peanut	Slightly heavy, nutty; may "flash" at high temperature	Excellent in Oriental stir-fries, Thai and Indonesian dishes; also good for salads
Safflower	Fairly bland; good for frying since it does not foam; general use	Good for frying, sautéing, salad dressings, baking; use to dilute stronger oils and in mayonnaise
Sesame	Toasted sesame has a rich, strong flavor, while untoasted is lighter, more bland	Use toasted in salad dressings, Oriental dishes; untoasted for stir-fries
Soy	Bold if unrefined; high smoke point; general use	Used commercially in margarine and mayonnaise
Sunflower	Nearly tasteless and odorless; all-purpose	Good in salad dressings, stir-fries, mayonnaise; use for frying, sautéing, and to dilute stronger oils
Walnut	Silky, rich, mildly nutty; low smoke point	Excellent for sautéing and in salad dressings, pasta, potato and chicken salads

a percentage of their menu items so that they fall within the Healthy Dining guidelines: fresh fruits and vegetables, whole grains, lean proteins, and the best fats. These guidelines are so similar to THM that I felt instantly simpatico with every person connected to Healthy Dining. The event brought together thirty restaurants from the San Diego area, presenting their best dishes. I tasted beautiful things that afternoon that were vibrant, flavorful, and so life giving I thought to myself, "Why can't we eat this kind of food in restaurants all the time? Why isn't this standard fare?" One of my favorite concepts, which was discussed throughout the afternoon, was the idea of encouraging your family to eat five fruits and vegetables a day. I had heard of this before, of course, but hearing so many people in one room committed to it made me take this bit of advice home to my children. Since that day, I have been trying to always make sure my kids and I eat our five fruits and vegetables before we can have pleasure food. Often when I tell people that I am trying to do this with everyone in my family (including myself), they laugh and say, "I can't even think of five fruits and vegetables that my kids will eat."

When I decided to write this book, one of the things I set out to prove to myself is that every child, regardless of how old he is or where he lives, has five favorite fruits and five favorite vegetables. I polled kids from all over the country by sending surveys to schools in Boston, Chicago, and Los Angeles, asking for each child's five favorite foods, five favorite fruits, and five favorite vegetables. There was not one survey that didn't mention at least five, and very often more than five, especially in the fruit department. I keep going back to one of the main themes of this book, "If you build it, they will come." I guarantee that if you stock your refrigerator with your child's favorite fruits and vegetables, she will eat at least five of them every day. You have to be creative, but this is the best way I know how to get your children to eat the most nutrient-dense foods we have. My advice, of course, is to make it organic produce because organic tastes so much better, even though it's not always as pretty as supermarket fruit. You may end up spending a little more money buying organic, but there's nothing more expensive than throwing away uneaten, tasteless fruits and vegetables (except for maybe bad health!).

Suggestions for Introducing New Fruits and Vegetables

We polled kids across the United States between the ages of two and a half to eighteen and found the top ten favorite fruits and vegetables for each age group. Below are the results, as well as twenty-five other suggestions to try. For age-specific favorites, please see Chapters 9 to 13.

Top Ten Fruits and Vegetables

Top Ten Fruits	*Top Ten Vegetables*
Apple	Carrots
Banana	Broccoli
Orange	Cucumbers
Strawberries	Lettuce
Grapes	Peas
Pineapple	Corn
Watermelon	Green beans
Peaches	Celery
Cantaloupe	Potato
Cherries	Spinach

Twenty-Five Fruits and Vegetables to Try

Fruits to try	*Vegetables to try*
Apricot	Artichoke
Blackberries	Arugula
Blood orange	Asparagus
Blueberries	Avocado
Cherimoya	Beet
Clementine	Bok choy
Crenshaw	Broccoli stems—raw and peeled
Figs	Brussels sprouts
Grapefruit	Cabbage, red
Guava	Cauliflower

Fruits to try	*Vegetables to try*
Honeydew	Collard greens
Kiwi	Cucumbers—small pickling ones peeled
Kumquat	Daikon radish
Lychee	Eggplant
Mango	Green and red pepper— sliced raw, roasted
Nectarine	Jicama
Papaya	Parsnip
Passion fruit	Radicchio
Pear	Red leaf lettuce
Plums	Romaine lettuce
Pomegranate	Rutabaga
Raspberries	Summer squash
Star fruit	Sweet potato
Tangelo	Turnip
Tangerine	Zucchini—julienne, grilled

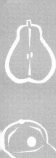

5

············

So How Do We Help Them?

Creating a Healthy Relationship Between Food and Hunger

How to Read Your Child's Appetite Signals

We have already discussed in Chapter 3 the concept of avoiding the use of food as a comfort, reward, or punishment. We already know that it is best not to automatically soothe our child with food anytime she gets hurt. But what about those times when she is crying or whining for something, and we are not sure what it is, so we give her food just to appease her or to keep her quiet? How do we know when our child is truly hungry, and not just tired, or thirsty, or needing exercise, or plain old bored? Later on in the book we will discuss recognizing an infant's cries as the real call of hunger, but what about our older kids, who seem to be out of control and acting out? We think that calming them down with food is just what the doctor ordered.

You usually know when your children have eaten and what they've eaten at mealtimes, but many times kids will say that they are hungry when they're really not. Saying "I'm hungry!" has become the thing kids do as a conditioned response to any uncomfortable feeling in order to buy time to figure out what they really want. (This is especially used as a stall tactic before going to bed.) The conditioned response works both ways. Kids are conditioned to say, "I'm hungry," which can mean "I'm bored," "I'm tired," or "I'm thirsty." Parents are conditioned to gratify this squawking without further investigation just to get them to quiet down. I can't tell you the number of times I've seen parents (my own included) try to calm down a noisy herd of kids with some sugary, fat-laden treat, only to regret it twenty minutes later when the noisy herd stampeded. I have found through my years of parenting and stepparenting that most of the time when children are misbehaving or whining, it's usually because they need to do something physical. Just as an adult always feels better after working out and breaking a sweat, so does a child. I think the one phrase I heard most as a kid was my mother telling one of us, "Run around the block a couple of times!" She knew that with six kids, when we would go at each other it usually meant we had been in the house too long and needed to let off steam running around. Next time one of your children says "I'm hungry," and you know he probably means something else, give him a glass of water first. Thirst is often mistaken for hunger. If that doesn't do the trick, then heed my mother's advice. It may not be safe to let him run around the block, but do try to get him engaged in some physical activity. He is probably bored or tired or restless and needs to get some oxygen in his system.

Physical activity usually works with all ages. There will be times, however, when your child may be hungry but it may be an emotional hunger due to the stress of peer pressure, schoolwork, and/or raging hormones. Our children (just like us) may want to eat not out of hunger, but out of the lack of control they feel somewhere else in their lives. There are many circumstances in a child's life that can trigger emotional eating, but it is up to us as parents to pay attention when this starts. You may want to check out your own habit of eating out of stress. Children pay attention to everything we do, even when we wish we weren't doing it.

Training a Palate

When your child is very, very young, the most important thing you have to remember is that his palate is not like yours. He hasn't spent years abusing it with salty, sugary, chemicalized foods. He is going to be a lot more sensitive to flavors than you are. I can't tell you how many parents taste the food they are going to give their infant and think it's too bland, so immediately they want to add salt and sugar to it. In fact, baby food companies for years added salt and sugar to punch up the flavors of natural fruit and vegetables. Fruits and vegetables, especially if they are organic, have enough flavor on their own.

The best thing you can do to train a palate is to avoid anything extreme—nothing too salty, nothing too sugary, nothing too spicy, and nothing with chemicals. If your child is older, start buying the healthier versions of whatever he likes, so that he won't continue tasting the strong, chemicalized flavorings in processed food, made not by God, but by the New Jersey Turnpike. We make jokes in my family all the time when we smell most brands of microwave popcorn or the food in food courts. We call it New Jersey Turnpike Popcorn or New Jersey on a Stick.

It may take a while, but your child will gradually appreciate the flavor of the healthier foods you give him.

There was a box of unopened healthy graham crackers languishing in the back of the cupboard for months. I figured my kids just didn't care for them. But now that the chocolate chip cookies, Oreos, and chips are gone, they are excited to get the plain graham crackers! I never would have thought that would happen.—ROSEMARY M. GUIDRY, MICHIGAN

Listening to Your Child's Body

When your child tells you that she doesn't like something or doesn't want something, sometimes you have to listen to what she is saying. Many times it is about a preferred flavor, but just as often, especially if she is very young, it can be about a food to which her body has a bad reaction. As a child, I did not like milk. I never felt good after drinking it, and the teachers at school were always trying to force it on me. The smell of cheese also bothered me. But once I got older, I got past my distaste for it and actually became addicted to it. Dairy became very difficult to give up, even after I learned the truth about it and even though eating it never made me feel good. You can get past an original distaste for a particular food that does not sit well with you. It can then cross over into addiction. People tend to become addicted to the things they are allergic to. I have people say to me all the time, "I could never give up sugar. I'm practically addicted to it," or, "I could never give up dairy. It's the only thing I like to eat." When I hear this, I know in all likelihood that person is allergic to the thing he most craves.

There are children who won't drink their milk or eat meat, or they don't like peanuts, and so on. If you hear that, chances are your child may have a reaction to it within his body that he cannot express in words. There is a story of an athlete who didn't want to drink milk as a child, but his father always challenged him to drink it. According to the father, it became a real contest of wills. When this athlete was a child, his body may have been trying to tell him something. As an asthmatic he probably naturally knew that he should not be eating dairy products.

Sometimes our kids know more than we do, or at least their systems are giving them information that we need to pay attention to. And I don't mean "I hate vegetables" or "I don't want dinner, I only want dessert." If a child has a true distaste for a particular food, it may be because he does not feel well after eating it. Many children have wheat allergies. Notice your child's temperament after eating wheat products. Does he seem out of control? Does he seem angry and short-tempered? Or tired and lethargic? Does his belly get a little swollen? That's one of the true signs of a wheat allergy. After eating dairy products, does your child have a stuffy nose, or does his throat feel thick and clogged? Does he have a hard time going to the bathroom? Is he a bed-wetter? That is a definite sign that your child may be allergic to dairy. If your child is completely out of control, nervous, and irritable and comes crashing down twenty minutes after eating sugar, I would remove as much sugar from his diet as you possibly can. And, of course, watch for all the chemicals in your child's food. Children who eat mostly processed foods have reactions and feel completely out of control.

Making the Transition from Unhealthy to Healthy Foods

One of the questions I get asked most is "How do I transition my child from unhealthy to healthy foods?" We have been eating the typical American diet for so long now, how do we get our children to appreciate the flavors of real food, as opposed to the oversugared, oversalted processed food that they are so used to? How do we get them to eat fruit instead of a candy bar, veggie burgers instead of hamburgers, and Knudsen Spritzers instead of Coca-Cola? It can be done at any age, but of course it is easier when they are younger. Children are naturally curious, and if you make a game out of getting healthy, your children will want to play. The first thing I will tell you is that if you are excited about getting healthy, your child will pick up your enthusiasm. But if you are saying, "Oh my gosh, this is going to be so difficult," it may come back to haunt you. She's not going to like getting healthy any more than you're going to like dragging her kicking and screaming to better health. But if you're excited about it, she will be, too.

Chemicals

First of all, get your kids in the habit of reading labels. Becoming aware of the chemistry in my food was the first of the ten steps I took to become healthy, and it is probably the most important one of all. As I always say, "You're a real person. Eat real food!" If you get your children in the habit of reading what they're eating, it will make a huge difference. If you or they can't pronounce it, chances are they should not be eating it. When my boys say, "Oh we want this!" I'll say, "Can you read it to me?" My son Nicky is a very good reader, and he knows that if he can't pronounce something, it's not going into his body. Children love going to the grocery store. In fact, kids love to do tasks we may hate because we do them so often. Can you think of anything more adorable than a five-year-old helping you wash clothes or make dinner? They're so enthusiastic; they love to learn, they love to do what you do. They even enjoy setting the table and doing the dishes. So take advantage of any of those chores that they want to do at those early ages. Get them involved in grocery shopping, and if they're too young to read labels, you can have them look for certain words or certain things. They can always count the number of ingredients. Chances are, if there are more than five ingredients, it's probably a processed food.

The goal, of course, is to eat whole foods that have no other ingredients but themselves. My advice is also to shop in a health food store. If you haven't been to one and won't know what you're looking at, it would probably be a good idea to go there and familiarize yourself with some of the products before you shop. I'm giving you the complete shopping list of kid-friendly foods at the end of this book. You may also want to check out Chapter 3 in my book *Healthy Life Kitchen*, in which I take you, aisle by aisle, shelf by shelf, to a Whole Foods Store and explain almost every item. Health food stores at first can be daunting, but if you familiarize yourself with the products, you will soon find that the food tastes so much better than what you get at a regular grocery store. The real whole flavor of whole food will make such a difference that soon your palate won't want anything else. After changing your palate to healthy foods, any food that has chemicals and preservatives in it will taste metallic and fake. When shopping in any store, remember it is always best to shop the perimeter as much as possible. That is where most of the whole foods are. Fruits and vegetables, fish, eggs, juices, and so on can all be bought there. It's those inner aisles, with their packaged goods, that will do the most damage.

My kids have been sick a lot this year with chronic ear infections. I suggested that we eliminate dairy and chemicals from our diet. I have already noticed an improvement in their health, and as a bonus their behavior has also improved. I wouldn't suggest that you do everything at once, but pick one or two steps and do them with commitment so your child can see the benefit for himself. Little by little I started eliminating all foods in our house that had "illegal" ingredients. It was a lot but I gave it all to our local food bank so I didn't feel so bad about getting rid of so much food. It was so much easier when all the bad stuff was not hanging around.—DEBORAH MCCLOSKEY, MARILU.COM

I began THMing this August. I read your book in one weekend. It hugely impacted me. To discover your books was a godsend. I have 2 children, ages 4 and 2. I have two tips. One—buy whole, unprocessed "snack" foods. Two—clean out your pantries and refrigerators and get rid of everything processed and full of chemicals.—ANDREA YOLAR, CALIFORNIA

Sugar

Refined sugar is one of the easiest health robbers to wean your children off of because there are so many treats that you can buy at a health food store—delicious goodies that are made with the "legal" sugars: raw honey, barley malt, fruit juice, maple syrup, maple sugar, Sucanat, stevia, Rapidura, raw cane juice, and agave. These sugars have not been put through a process that removes all of the nutrients. They will definitely give you an energy boost, but not so high that you will come crashing down twenty minutes later feeling awful the way sugar does. These treats taste like the so-called real thing, but won't make your kids crazy. I know it's hard to believe, but if your children start eating more real food and more centered food, you will be amazed at how their craving for sweets of any kind (even the legal ones) will decrease. The best way to start weaning your children off refined sugar is to stop buying it for your house.

If you are a truly sugar-addicted family, go to the health food store and stock your house with legal treats that the kids will enjoy, no matter how big their sweet tooth is. I dare anyone to taste an Uncle Eddie's Vegan Cookie (chocolate chip or peanut butter–chocolate chip, especially) and not think it tastes as good or better than what they are used to. These cookies are my favorite treats to bring whenever someone says, "Healthy desserts never have enough flavor for me." What's great about these cookies is that their taste is unforgettable, but you'll only want one or two. Legal treats will satisfy your sweet tooth, but keep you off that sugar treadmill that so many sugar treats put you on.

My four-year-old had a trip with his preschool to Candyland, where they made their own candy treats for Easter. He came home with 3 chocolate pops that he made all by himself. He asked me if they were in his "diet." I told him that they weren't and I listed the various ingredients that were probably in them (milk, sugar, food coloring . . .). He looked so disappointed. I said to him, "You know we are all trying to be healthy but I will let you decide what you want to do." He is 4 years old; of course he ate one. Within twenty minutes he was buckled over in pain in the bathroom telling me his tummy hurt. Then he said, "Mommy, we should have just thrown the candy in the trash!" What a painful but great lesson.—DEBORAH MCCLOSKEY, MARILU.COM

Meat

When I gave up meat twenty-two years ago, there were very few substitutes for beef. Nowadays you can get anything you want in any form or flavor that you want, based on turkey or chicken or fish or soy products. The spices that are added to these alternatives will taste so much like the foods you grew up with that you'll be convinced you're still eating them. In other words, you don't have to give up your burgers, your Sloppy Joes, or your meatballs, because every single dish can be duplicated, but with healthier ingredients than beef or pork. One of my favorite things to eat as a child was breakfast sausage, and for years after giving up meat, I missed that flavor. Now, however, since Yves' and Amy's and Boca Burgers have been on the scene, I don't miss my sausages. These brands use soy and, with the right spices, take me back to Sunday morning breakfast with the family. Most of the dishes we make with ground beef are really about the seasoning or condiments. If you dress up a veggie burger with ketchup, mustard, relish, tomato, onions, lettuce, and pickle, your brain will tell you that you are eating the real thing. Meatloaf and Sloppy Joes are really about what tomato sauce or ketchup or vegetables you put on them. So you can add your special sauce to ground turkey meat or textured soy protein and fool even your biggest meat eaters. If you are trying to wean your family off beef and pork products and are not ready to become completely vegan, try Shelton Farms turkey and chicken products. Their products are preservative free and made from free-range poultry meat.

The health food store will open up a whole new world for you in terms of meat substitutes. This past year, while traveling around the country, I found a Whole Foods grocery store in almost every city. If you are fortunate enough to have one in your area, check out the meat substitutes not only in the refrigerators, but also at the meat counter. There you can find hot dogs, sausages, and other meat products made from turkey, chicken, fish, and even vegetables that will make you think you are in an old-fashioned butcher shop. With all of the panic surrounding foot-and-mouth and mad cow disease, it's good to know that you don't have to sacrifice your health for flavor anymore!

I was a hamburger, French fry and coffee frappe, steak and potato, lamb chop girl. One of the first things I did was give up meat. I was surprised how easy it was for me. I found healthy substitutes. If I felt like a steak, I would have some swordfish, and if I feel like a burger, I reach for a vegan Boca Burger or a portobello mushroom cap burger. I find that satisfies my "craving" and is a much healthier alternative. I also found I don't crave it as much as I thought I would after giving it up. As for free-range chicken, it is the only chicken I buy now. It tastes better and isn't yellow like other grocery brands. We eat chicken once a week as well as fish once a week. The other five meals I try to make vegetarian for our family.—MARILU.COM USER

Dairy

Once you have made the commitment to give up dairy products, you will realize how easy it is to make so many of your favorite dishes with a milk substitute. Product by product, you can find a healthy alternative that will not only taste good but will also make you feel better because your nose won't be stuffy, your throat won't be phlegmy, and your digestion will be greatly improved (and you know what that means!). Anyone who has ever read any of my books knows that I was very addicted to dairy products for a long period of time. In fact, giving up dairy was the hardest of the ten steps I took to become healthy. I was obsessed with dairy and would eat it every day. When it was first suggested to me that I give up dairy to improve my health, I said, "There's no way I'm going to give up my cheese, my milk, my yogurt," and everything else I used to love eating. I'm here to tell you that if you make the commitment to give up dairy products to improve your health, you will never regret it. If there's one step that everyone who tries the Total Health Makeover program talks about, it is how giving up dairy has changed her life.

Product by product, there is a healthy alternative. For milk, the two that are most highly recommended are Original Enriched Rice Dream by Imagine Foods and Silk Soy Milk, original flavor, by White Wave. The latter is a great milk substitute for cooking. As I have already mentioned, Earth Balance Margarine is the best butter substitute because it has no hydrogenated oils in it. For a cheese substitute, the Lite n' Less Veggie Singles by Soyco are my family's favorite, especially for grilled cheese sandwiches. There are substitutes for sour cream, cream cheese, and even a soy cream to replace half-and-half. And for yogurt, I dare anyone to taste a Whole Soy brand yogurt and not think it is better than the one they are used to eating.

Sometimes you have to be crafty with your family. (Not dishonest, of course, just a little crafty!) As I always suggest to people who are starting out, add rice milk or soy milk, a little at a time, to your children's milk, beginning with one-quarter rice or soy, three-quarters cow's milk. Gradually increase the percentage of rice or soy milk until that's all your children are drinking. Basically you are weaning them off the flavor of cow's milk. Interestingly enough, most people, after giving it up, dislike the flavor of cow's milk if they ever "cheat" and taste it again. I always explain to people that on this program there is no such thing as cheating. It is just checking your progress to see how far you've come. If you cook some of the recipes in this book, I guarantee your children will not taste the difference from conventional foods, especially if you start by putting a limited amount of dairy in your food. You know your family, so you'll know if they are a cold turkey family or the kind that has to be weaned. Cold turkey might be hard for some. If you go that route, I suggest giving up dairy products for a few weeks before you start substituting with soy cheese. The milk is an easier substitution because Original

Enriched Rice Dream, for example, tastes like the milk after you've eaten your cereal. So many people have been successful with weaning their family off dairy products that I think I will let a testimonial speak for itself.

I was a bit sneaky when it came to turning the family over to THM. I would buy organic cereals that were "legal" and I would never tell them. I would also mix the milk—half soy milk and half regular milk. After a while I would increase the soy to the point where I would no longer add milk. Milk was then no longer purchased. I would buy Roma coffee for my husband and he still does not miss his Folgers. It took a year but I think they finally cleansed their palates. My husband went from 195 lbs. to 164 lbs. since the change, so he's not complaining. My family had to slowly make the adjustment, but now we're all THMers. My kids just assume that I'm buying them the same old stuff that I used to buy. Once the kids were eating healthy foods and eliminating the junk foods—the doctor didn't see them much for a while!! My friends sometimes crack a joke about my "weird" eating habits and how I can sometimes "deprive" my children of the good things in life by having them on this program, but it goes in one ear and out the other. My children are healthy, and I mean REALLY healthy!!—Janet Van Ess, Wisconsin

Eating Outside the Home

Restaurant Techniques

Once you have decided to set up this fabulous world of health for your child at home, it's easy to practice the same principles in the outside world, as long as you plan ahead and adopt some healthy tactics. You won't have as much control over your child's diet as you do at home, but by learning how to read a menu and carrying some of your own staples with you, you can make eating healthy outside the home as convenient as possible. And when it's not, you can always rest assured that as long as your child is receiving the best food possible at home, eating something unhealthy in the outside world can always be compensated for later in your kitchen.

One of the lessons I have learned from taking my children to restaurants is this: don't let your kids order anything with sugar in it. It will instantly make your child's blood sugar rise, and you may have a child who is more hyper at the table than you want him to be. Be careful with fruit juice as well. The only time I give my kids fruit juice is when we find ourselves in a restaurant later than their usual dinner time and I want them to stay up. Even then, I make sure to cut the fruit juice in half with sparkling water, and I give them only 100 percent natural fruit juice. This will keep them a little more awake, but not bouncing off the walls like a Shirley Temple would (and the chemicals in the maraschino cherries don't help!).

I have also learned the hard way that I do not want them to be filling up on the white flour bread usually found in the bread basket. If they do eat some bread, I try to make it whole grain as often as possible, and they eat it not with butter, but rather olive oil and a little balsamic vinegar. I know it may sound a little LA to some people, but my kids actually do like olive oil with a splash of balsamic vinegar. Sure they like the flavor, but they really like the art designs the separation creates. We definitely get the butter off the table, not only because we don't eat it, but also because at this point we can't even stand the smell of it. One of the best things I've learned when taking my kids to restaurants is to give them soup first. They're usually thirsty when they first sit down, and soup is nice and wet. Besides, it is a great way to get them to eat their vegetables. And it's also a great way of slowing down the eating time so they're not finishing their entire meal before the rest of the table has gotten their entrees. Kids will actually learn to dine with their parents as long as we take the time to dine with *them*. My kids have been eating in restaurants since they were very young because I have always loved eating in restaurants. Some of my best memories from childhood are eating in restaurants with my parents and I wanted my kids to have that same experience.

Get Your Child Moving

If you have read my book *The 30-Day Total Health Makeover*, you may remember that what I recommend when you're creating an exercise program for you, the grown-ups, is to rediscover the child within yourself and have FUN! Well, your child is already a child so getting her to move should be easy. The key word is "fun." Whether you're old or young, you will not enjoy exercising, or stay with it, unless you are having fun doing it. This is even more important for kids. Here are a few suggestions:

◆ Instead of buying your children another video game for their birthdays or Christmas, how about a basketball, soccer ball, tennis racket, baseball, jump rope, or any other kind of sporting equipment that may just spark something. Pick the sport that *you* are most likely to join.

◆ Take the time to teach them a physical activity that you know. Kids enjoy sports and activities much more when they excel at them. So be creative and teach them well. They just might get really good at something they'll enjoy the rest of their lives. Think of how proud you'll be when Junior dedicates his ESPY award to you.

◆ Stay involved in your child's physical education classes at school. Ask about frequency of classes and activity, class size, curriculum. Show his PE teachers that you care by getting to know them. Don't be shy about asking the teachers what kind of program they follow and what their philosophy is concerning children's fitness.

◆ Get your child involved in team sports. This can teach him the importance of teamwork and help him cope with peer pressure.

◆ Sign them up for lessons. If there's no class, check the phonebook or sign up at your local Y or recreation center. Maybe you could even take a class together. Even though they don't always act like it, kids really enjoy doing sports and recreation much more when they do it with Mom and Dad.

◆ Don't allow anything after school except homework or exercise or practicing a musical instrument—no television, video games, or junky snacks.

◆ For younger kids, avoid strollers and playpens as much as possible. Allow them the freedom to move, but make sure that they are always safe.

If your kids look bored, make suggestions that get them moving: spud, dodgeball, volleyball, iceskating, or building a snowman. You can even play "follow the leader" around the house if they're stuck indoors.

Creating an Exercise Habit That Will Last a Lifetime

Try to get your child involved in one sport in which he will remain interested. When a child enjoys a particular sport, he is likely to stay with it for years, perhaps a lifetime, and reaps the healthy physical and mental rewards that come with that. So, go ahead, and invest in dance lessons, tennis lessons, basketball, or karate. If he quits (and sometimes children do), don't make a big deal out of it or he might not want to try something else later. Hang in there. The next endeavor may be the one that changes his life. I have always felt lucky because when I was growing up, my family owned a dancing school. I have been dancing since I was four years old. I have always loved to move as a result, and even when I weighed 174 pounds (before I created THM, of course), I could always cut a rug on the dance floor. Having a body that has been used to some kind of physical activity since childhood made it that much easier for me to get into shape once I really got serious about exercise. It was as if my body had been computerized to sweat and tone in childhood, and as an adult, I just had to "reboot" the program.

Movement is not only essential for a healthy body, it also does wonders for a child's mind. Physical therapist Ted Pastrick explains:

INCORPORATING MOVEMENT INTO LEARNING

Children need movement in order to learn. Movement is an essential component because it allows them to explore their environment. They don't need to understand it on an intellectual level. They don't need to see it written down. They need to do it! When we move, we're using not only our muscles but also our whole sensory system: vision, balance, and proprioception (this tells us the position of our limbs in relation to each other and the environment). So movement is a way of increasing one's learning ability because our nervous system has these built-in systems. As a baby develops, the first system that gets completely wired and ready for use is the vistibular system, which deals with balance and hearing. Movement challenges that system constantly. If a baby is crawling on all fours and she picks up one hand, for instance, there are receptors in the semicircular canals of her ear that are sensing where her head is in space. It is sending that information to her brain, and the brain is creating networks of connections as a result of that movement. Her brain is actually being stimulated to grow as a result of that movement. Movement is a way of developing a child's nervous system. And the nervous system grows not just in relationship to intellectual information, or conceptual information, but also in relationship to where it is physically. What is its physical state in the world? If we were plants, we couldn't move. Our whole system would be different. But we have legs and we move in order to explore the world. So that ability to move and explore the world feeds into the intellectual world. We understand more about the world because of this movement. The more we bring our whole sensory system into a learning experience, the better our understanding will be of that experience. Imagine the difference in a child's understanding of a lemon when we compare a child merely seeing a photograph of a lemon to actually holding it, feeling it, catching it, squeezing it, smelling it, and tasting it.

Similarly, my sons' PE teacher, Susan Cole, uses some wonderful games to incorporate movement and exercise into her lessons about diet and nutrition. The following is one example:

We throw a bunch of pictures of various foods out in the schoolyard, and then tell the children to pick up their favorite food or whichever food they can get their hands on. After they've made their choice, they turn the picture over and read the amount of exercise they'll have to do in order to burn the fat and calories contained in the food they chose. All the kids who pick pizza, burgers, candy, or other junk foods have to run around the schoolyard several times. All the kids who pick up fruits or vegetables only have to do a little exercise, but they still have to do some. I try to get the point across that exercise is necessary even if we eat healthy food. This is a great lesson. It gets the point across and the kids remember, too. The second time we play it, the kids invariably rush to pick up the healthy foods.

—SUSAN COLE, PE TEACHER

MOTIVATING AN OVERWEIGHT CHILD

The best way to inspire children to move and exercise is to create the opportunity for them to do what they're able to do in a way that they'll enjoy. Kids will not do anything consistently unless they enjoy it. Parents often make the mistake of sizing up what they themselves believe is the problem with their child—obesity, inactivity, junk food, etc. After they've identified the problem, they independently determine a plan of action and impose this plan, often against the will of the child. This creates the perfect environment for conflict, struggle, disappointment, failure for both, and ultimately, a wider gap in parent-child understanding. Often it takes a while for parents to disinvest in the set of rules that they originally planned for the child.

You have to relate to every child on an individual basis and put in what I call due diligence by really observing what your child gets excited about. This has nothing to do with what you think is exciting or the perfect solution. Some kids are highly motivated by competition and some are not. Some kids are driven to succeed; others couldn't care less. If your child gets excited about anything at all that has to do with movement, go with that. But you have to be subtle in your encouragement. If you go overboard and say, "Okay, let's do it! This is great! This is going to be just the thing to get you thin and healthy!" you create pressure. He'll feel like he's being manipulated and that you're stepping on his song. Children need to do things for themselves. They need to take personal pride in their activities. Backing off is one of the hardest things for a parent to do. Parents are often invested in some sort of image that they are imposing on their child. A big problem for kids is dealing with the egos of their parents.

You have to observe your child and look at what she really likes and encourage that. For example, if she likes Ping-Pong, but you feel she needs more exercise than what she's getting from Ping-Pong, you should instead step back a bit and say privately to yourself, "Ping-Pong will get her moving somewhat and she enjoys it. That's great!" And you should do this without your child being aware that you have energy on it. This is very difficult to do. You really have to walk a fine line here. You have to do this on their terms, not yours.—TED PASTRICK, M.P.T.

Healthy Tips to Live By

✦ When you go grocery shopping, don't buy the temptation foods to begin with. Try to exercise your strongest willpower when you're shopping. Keep the naughty stuff out of sight and it will automatically be out of mind.

✦ Decrease your family's fat intake. This is getting easier since there are so many lower fat choices of foods available. But be careful and read every label because many low fat foods are high in sugar, sodium, and chemicals. Have you ever noticed that the larger "LOW FAT" is written on the label, the more that product tends to sneak in other health robbers to enhance its flavor or shelf-life. Also, an excess of low fat foods can lead to weight gain, too.

✦ Limit or completely eliminate fast foods.

✦ When dining out, pick healthier choices from the adult menu, rather than limiting their choices to the kid's menu. Have them share an appetizer and/or entree. The kid's menu is often filled with choices high in fat, sodium, and sugar.

✦ Allow your taste buds to reacquaint themselves with food in its purest form (whole foods). You'll start to have a renewed appreciation for live foods. Live foods really do taste better.

✦ Try to serve your children five servings of fruits and vegetables and a generous amount of whole grains every day.

✦ For the next week or so, keep track of all foods you and your family consume. Make a list with two columns. One column for all the whole foods and the other for processed foods. Get ready. This can be a real eye opener for some people.

✦ Fun little pleasure foods can still be part of your family's health, but you have to be more conscious of them.

✦ Allow your kids to complain about "health food" rather than give in to poor eating habits. This is much better in the long run for their health and your sanity.

✦ The first choice for fruits and vegetables should be whatever is grown somewhat locally, in season, and organic, if possible.

✦ Frequently boil or steam a medium or large size bowl of soybeans (edemame). This makes a great between-meal snack for the family.

✦ Try to serve your kids at least one cup of beans and/or legumes daily. It lowers serum cholesterol about 10 percent after twenty-one days.

✦ Never use food as a reward.

✦ Kids don't want to dine. They like foods that are easy to handle like finger foods and things you can eat on the go and all of the other cute foods that belong to the world of childhood. Convert healthy foods so they have the look, feel, and convenience of fun, snacky, kids' foods. Keep a bowl of fruit and a bowl of vegetables cut up and ready to go in the fridge, especially for after school. Think about what would make healthy food appealing to your children. Be creative.

✦ Introduce a new fruit or vegetable every week that your family has never or rarely eaten. Most people are surprised when they learn about all the wonderful varieties there are out there.

✦ Get your kids in the habit of reading labels. This is a great way to become aware of the chemicals and additives that are in many of our foods.

✦ The best way to start weaning your children off refined sugar is to stop buying it for your house. If your family sugar addiction has been fairly serious, go to the health food store and stock your house with legal treats that the kids will enjoy no matter how big their sweet tooth is.

✦ Introduce new foods gradually, especially for really young kids. Offer the child a small portion but do not force him to eat it or put too much energy on it. Developing a fondness for some foods occasionally takes a while. If you push too hard the first time, they may never like it.

✦ Get your kids involved in planning, shopping, reading labels, and cooking.

✦ Make sure the portions you serve are reasonable.

✦ Explore the world of meat substitutes. You'll find great flavors that are easy on your digestive system.

✦ The key word for exercise is "fun." Whether you're old or young, you will not enjoy exercising, or stay with it, unless you are having fun doing it.

✦ Frequently plan fun physical activities for the whole family.

✦ Limit television, computer, and video game time.

✦ You have to relate to every child on an individual basis and put in what I call due diligence by really observing what kind of physical activity your child gets excited about.

✦ Encourage and find physical activities that your children really enjoy. Be creative here. This can be fun! It's amazing how something as silly as a Ping-Pong table can change a child's life.

✦ There are many things in a child's life that can trigger emotional eating, but it is up to us as parents to pay attention when this starts. You may want to check out your own habit of eating out of stress. Children pay attention to everything we do, even when we wish we weren't doing it.

✦ The first thing you have to understand, especially if your child is under five years old, is that her palate is different from yours.

✦ Don't allow snacking in the car, in front of the television, or while doing homework. Studies show that eating in front of the television is a major contributor to weight problems.

✦ Do not allow your kids to have a television in their rooms. There is absolutely no reason for that, and it inspires laziness and mindless snacking.

✦ Monitor the school lunch program. If you don't like what you see, encourage more packed lunches.

✦ Help kids become aware of their own feelings of hunger and fullness. This starts with learning to distinguish a baby's "I am hungry" cry from other cries. There will be times when you will allow your baby second or third helpings of some foods, and other times when it's important not to force one more bite.

✦ Kids learn most by example. Adopt a healthy lifestyle, and odds are your children will, too. Eat junk and you can be sure your children will, too.

✦ Be enthusiastic about eating a variety of foods. Help children understand the different food groups and why it's important to eat some of each group daily.

✦ If children are overweight before adolescence, the goal is to try to maintain the same weight. This way, as children gain in height, they will thin out. Prevention is the key. Keep track of your child's height and weight throughout childhood. This will help identify children at risk.

✦ Never put a child on a weight reduction diet. This teaches him to ignore feelings of hunger and may lead him to believe there is truly something wrong with him for wanting to eat more. A child often perceives it as a form of punishment.

✦ Don't calorie-restrict children. Don't obsess with your child over every fat gram and sugar calorie or take dieting, low fat, or no fat eating to the extreme. The goal is to make better choices and establish a normal eating pattern.

Now that you are armed with knowledge and a game plan, how do you address your child's specific needs? Every age comes with a unique set of circumstances as well as obstacles to overcome. The following chapters are meant to give you solutions to some of the challenges your child faces within his particular age group.

6

· · · · · · · · · · · · ·

Breast-feeding

> **B**reast-fed babies' IQs are three to five points higher than those of formula-fed babies, according to a new report in the *American Journal of Clinical Nutrition*, which compiled the results of 11 previous studies and adjusted for factors that could affect results, such as parental intelligence or income. Breast-fed babies also showed more rapid maturation of visual and motor systems and fewer behavioral problems. The benefits are thought to be due to the type of fats in breast milk, which are somewhat different from those in cow's milk formulas. An IQ benefit has also been demonstrated with vegetarian diets.
>
> *Good Medicine*, vol. 9, no. 1 (Winter 2000)

When I first became pregnant with Nicky almost eight years ago, the big question expectant moms were asking themselves was whether or not they should breast-feed. This has changed. There has been a sharp increase in the percentage of women who are breast-feeding in the last thirty years, and especially in the last ten. Only about 25 percent of women in the United States breast-fed their babies in 1973 when breast-feeding was at an all-time low. Today it's about 67 percent and it has increased 20 to 25 percent (depending on which part of the country you are talking about) in the last decade. The reason for this dramatic change is a heightened awareness, which has rapidly spread in this country, of the enormous benefits of breast-feeding.

It is recommended that a child breast-feeds for at least one year of life, with solid foods not starting until six months of age. If this is the case, your baby stands a fighting chance to be healthy.—PETER S. WALDSTEIN, M.D., F.A.A.P.

The highest breast-feeding rates are among higher-income, college-educated women over thirty years old who are more likely than others to have access to information. We owe much to organizations like La Leche League, which offers mother-to-mother support, encouragement, information, and education, for disseminating this knowledge.

Benefits of Breast-feeding

Here are some of the benefits of breast-feeding:

+ Breast milk is nature's perfect food, fully capable of providing all the essential nutrients a baby needs up to the age of one.
+ During breast-feeding, the baby acquires antibodies from mom, which increases protection from numerous illnesses and diseases. Breast-fed babies get fewer colds and ear infections, and recover faster when they do.
+ Not only is the structure of breast milk perfect overall, it can change in composition based on a baby's needs at any given time. Day one milk is different from day seven, morning milk is different from afternoon, and one month is different from six months. No synthetic formula can change throughout the day, month, or year.
+ Breast-feeding creates a special bonding with mom, who receives health benefits of her own from the experience.
+ Breast milk has six to ten times more linolenic acid and other essential fatty acids than cow's milk. These fatty acids are the building blocks

for neurological development and delicate neuromuscular control in humans.

✦ Cow's milk is designed to build massive skeletal and muscle tissue. It is wonderfully designed for turning a 45-pound calf into a 300-pound cow in less than one year and has no business in the body of any human being, much less the delicate intestines of an infant.

✦ Breast milk protein is mostly lactalbumin, which is designed for a human baby's sensitive digestive system. Cow's milk protein is mostly casein, which is likely to cause spitting up, gas, and colic.

✦ Breast milk puts less stress on a baby's kidneys because it is lower in sodium and protein than cow's milk.

✦ Cow's milk has too much phosphorus, an excess of which interferes with the absorption of calcium. So even though cow's milk has more calcium, breast milk utilizes it better.

✦ Allergies resulting from breast-feeding are very rare, and when they do occur, it is almost always because of something the mother ate and passed on to the baby. Ironically, this happens frequently when the mother consumes *cow's milk.*

✦ Breast-fed babies have a lower risk of heart disease in adulthood. Studies have shown that breast-fed babies have lower cholesterol on average as adults.

✦ Breast-fed babies suffer fewer bouts with diaper rash.

✦ Some evidence suggests that breast-feeding reduces the risk of breast cancer for some moms.

✦ Some research has revealed that breast-fed babies scored 3 to 5 points higher on IQ tests than babies nursed with cow's milk–based formula.

✦ Breast milk is a lot cheaper than any other choice. You don't need a calculator to figure this one out.

Wow! As you can see, the benefits are overwhelming. It's pretty one-sided, isn't it? You're probably wondering why so many women over the years (especially during the '60s and '70s) have chosen bottle-feeding over breast-feeding. There are a few reasons for this. Some women don't have a choice, and that's a reality. Other reasons are very subjective. One argument I've actually read in favor of bottle-fed cow's milk is that breast milk is easily digested and cow's milk is very difficult for a baby to digest. Believe it or not, some people consider this an advantage because it gives a baby a full and more satisfied feeling much longer. (I guess this is just like when an adult eats a cheeseburger and milkshake and usually doesn't get hungry again for several hours.) The same thing is true when a baby consumes cow's milk formula, but it puts a great burden on a baby's digestive system. Another so-called advantage to bottle-feeding, according to some people, is that it can be precisely measured, and a mom can feel comforted knowing her baby is consuming a so-called required amount. However, this is actually a disadvantage because a mother may assume she knows the correct or necessary amount her baby needs, but a baby's needs change throughout the day and throughout the month. The most natural amount a baby needs is best known by the baby herself, not by what her mother thinks is best. Babies instinctively know what they need, and during breast-feeding, they know exactly when to stop feeding. With bottle-feeding, the milk is basically poured in, like gas into a gas tank. When you list all of the so-called advantages of bottle-feeding (convenience, no fashion constraints, less conflict with work or free time, less concern about mom's diet, no public embar-rassment, no conflict with lovemaking), you realize that every advantage is really a disadvantage for the baby and that bottle-feeding could be perceived as a selfish choice on the part of the parents. How important are your baby's first six months of life (her most important developmental period) as opposed to these six months in your life?

When it came to breast-feeding, there was never any doubt in my mind. My mother breast-fed all six of us kids, which was somewhat unpopular during the '40s and '50s. Only about 1 in 3 moms breast-fed during that time. I remember watching my mom nursing my brother Lorin when I was five. Even at that age I thought it was wonderful. She seemed to be having such a positive experience. Not only did she exude a glow of loving, nurturing mom, she, oddly enough, often talked about how breast-feeding actually helped her regain her figure. She wasn't wrong. Breast-feeding helps shrink the uterus back to its normal size.

Okay, I think we are all pretty much in agreement here that breast-feeding is the way to go. Even the federal government is strongly encouraging women to breast-feed. U.S. Surgeon General David Satcher and the Department of Health and Human Services set a goal to significantly increase by the year 2010 the percentage of women who breast-feed their babies during year one of their child's life.

These days, nearly every mom wants to breast-feed her child; the problem is that not every woman is able to. Babies often never take to breast-feeding to begin with. And sadly, many babies who initially do take to it, reject it soon after. Many women go into the experience of motherhood planning to breast-feed but give up when they are faced with a crying baby, not enough information, and a free formula sample from the hospital. Currently, about 67 percent of new mothers in the United States start out breast-feeding their newborns, and by six months that number already drops to 30 percent. On one hand, I want to passionately encourage women to go out there and breast-feed, but on the other, I am fearful that many women will feel very sad if it turns out that they can't.

I want to address this issue in two ways. First, I want moms whose breast-feeding plans don't go quite the way they wanted them to go to remember that most people in the last two generations (Boomers and X'ers) were not breast-fed. (I know that this notion is a little scary considering some of the characters who came out of those two generations, but for the most part, we're all pretty normal.) Second, and this is very important, there are many choices a pregnant woman or new mom can make to stack the deck for successful full-term breast-feeding way in her favor.

If breast-feeding, after putting in your best effort, is not successful, keep in mind that there are some wonderful formulas out there. Also remember that there are some horrible formulas, too, ones that are full of preservatives and other questionable ingredients. Obviously I don't recommend any formulas that have cow's milk or ingredients like nonfat milk solids. I've known many babies who spit up frequently on cow's milk–based formula because they were allergic. But there are healthy formulas out there that are terrific and kids are just fine on them. Look especially into the ones that are soy-based (ProSoBee and Isomil). However, before you do go to formula, please learn as much as you can to increase your chances for successful breast-feeding.

It's Your Baby!

Why is it that some babies latch on and others don't? Why is it that some women find it so difficult to breast-feed and others find it to be as natural as a cat with her litter of kittens? I was obsessed with these questions long before my own pregnancies and did extensive research on the subject while I was pregnant. Perhaps the most important information I found was in several nonconventional books. They said that it's very important to put your baby to your breast immediately after birth, when natural sucking instinct is strongest. This might not seem like a big deal, but it can be crucial to the success of the breast-feeding over the first six to twelve months. If a baby doesn't suckle right away, he may not get another urge to do so for about forty-eight hours no matter how hard you try to get him to latch on. By that time he will have been fed formula in a bottle, which can easily become the baby's first choice, since it was the method of his first meal. That is why breast-feeding must be started before he does anything else, before the nurses take him away to be washed, measured, and weighed. I tried this with both of my boys and both of them latched on immediately. They were barely out of me before I put them on my breast. And they both took to it without any problems. I had an agreement with my doctor and the hospital before doing it this way. At the time it was not considered normal procedure. The problem for many moms is that most hospitals have very organized procedures that seem to be more concerned with hospital efficiency and speed than with the needs of the mother and child.

So it's very important that you create such a contract with your doctor long before your due date. Your doctor should know that it's your baby and give you what *you* want. And because you're the mother, you shouldn't let anyone talk you out of this. Start standing up for what's best for your child. Because of the volume of patients, hospital administrators want to make everything convenient for their staff. Luckily the system is changing somewhat because a lot of moms have been standing up for themselves and their babies.

In the old days, hospitals would immediately take your baby away, wash her measure her, put silver nitrate in her eyes, get her little footprint, and eventually get her spanking clean. How shocking this must have been for a newborn. It was also a way to get mom out of the room, get everything moved on, give the baby a bottle, and park her in the nursery with other babies. It was much easier for the hospital to keep all the babies in the same room and feed them with a bottle instead of carrying them all the way back to their mom when it was time to feed them. If babies are given bottles, especially in those first couple of days when it's so difficult for them to develop the skills that are necessary for suckling, the convenience of the bottle will keep them from adapting to the breast. That is why it is so important not to confuse a baby and give her a bottle in the early stages. Hospitals were, and some still are, concerned about the day or two that mother and child are spending with them and have little regard for the long-term effects their procedures could have on the mother and child's bonding and breast-feeding.

Establishing a Breast-feeding Pattern

If you really want your baby to stay with breast-feeding, you shouldn't give him a bottle for the first three weeks. The rule of thumb is usually three weeks before he should have any kind of bottle experience. Three weeks will establish enough of a breast-feeding pattern so that your baby won't want only a bottle if exposed to one. Then you will have the most successful breast-feeding relationship with your baby.

Position of the baby's mouth on the nipple is very important. Keep in mind that in order for your baby to extract milk effectively, his mouth should be surrounding and sucking on the areola, not the nipple. If your baby sucks only on the nipple, just a little milk will be released and the nipple will become easily irritated.

Breast-feeding is nature at its best. It is a wonderful and amazing supply-and-demand relationship between you and your child. Your baby's sucking stimulates nerve endings in your nipple, which sends a message to the pituitary gland in your brain to secrete two hormones: prolactin and oxytocin. A rapid increase of prolactin encourages milk production, and an increase of oxytocin causes the elastic tissue around the milk glands to contract, squeezing a large supply of milk through the milk ducts into the sinuses and out the nipple. It is one of nature's miracles. As long as this physical action is in play, your breasts will respond and continue to produce and expel milk. If your baby begins feeding less (perhaps because you are supplementing with formula or food), your body will respond by cutting back on milk production. Your body instinctively knows to produce more or less milk depending on your baby's needs. This supply-and-demand system allows mothers to produce enough milk for twins or even triplets. Using a pump will trick the breast somewhat, but nothing works like the natural stimulation and response that take place between mother and child. You can pump on average for about six weeks before your milk supply will decrease if you don't also have your baby himself feeding on the nipple. It's the baby's mouth and salivary glands that create that supply/demand relationship with the breast.

The wonderful complexity of breast-feeding is mind-boggling. Breast milk itself is not only the perfect food, with the precise amount of proteins, carbohydrates, and fats and enzymes, it is also uniquely designed for *your* child. While you carried your baby inside of you, your body instinctively created the right milk composition to feed your particular baby. And it continues to create the right composition after your baby leaves your body. Did you know that the consistency and makeup of breast milk actually changes depending on the weather? In very hot weather your breast milk has a higher water content, which is just what your baby needs.

They Are What You Eat

Keep in mind that during breast-feeding, what you yourself are eating is as important as ever because what you eat pretty much goes directly into your breast milk. This is the one time in your child's life when you are really in control of what she is eating. As long as you are eating healthy food, you can be confident that baby is, too. I've learned that it takes about eight hours to go from your mouth, at *your* mealtime, to your breasts for *his* mealtime. When people tell me their baby has been up all night, I'll ask them what they themselves ate the day before for lunch. Nine times out of ten it has been a big protein meal. If you have a big piece of fish for lunch, that high concentration of protein will reach your breasts at about eight or nine at night. Baby will get a big protein rush from breast-feeding just before bedtime. So plan your meals ahead of time. When you want your baby most awake, eat a protein meal eight or nine hours before. I had to completely readjust my starch meal or my protein meal to compensate for when I wanted my kids awake or asleep.

I learned the hard way about the "eight hours later" factor, or I should say Nicky learned the hard way. When he was two and half months old, I was passing my favorite Thai food restaurant one night and thought, "Oh, Thai food! I haven't had that since before I got pregnant!" Cut to the next morning. Nicky let out this bloodcurdling scream for no apparent reason and wouldn't stop crying for about ten minutes. I became really worried until I was finally able to calm him down, and then I did a little investigating. I thought to myself, "Could this have something to do with the Thai food I had last night for dinner?" I went and checked the breast milk supply I had pumped immediately after feeding Nicky that morning to see if it smelled like Thai food. Not only did it smell like Thai food, it had an oily red-chili-pepper-like residue floating on top. My poor baby! He was writhing in pain because he just had his first heavy dose of the famous number seven at Tommy Tang's—hot and spicy tom-ka-kai! It was his first number seven—but his worst number two. I did a little calculating. *His* mealtime was exactly eight hours after *my* mealtime. I remembered reading about the eight-hour turnaround and made the connection. After the tom-ka-kai incident, I based all of my meal planning on the eight-hour turnaround, but the big lesson of the day was NO MORE SPICY FOOD! It was July 26, 1994, and I wrote in Nicky's baby diary, "Today was the worst day of my life! Mommy decided to have Thai food!"

I think Nicky's first words were "NO MORE TOM-KA-KAI!"

Breast Milk: The Cure-All

But not to worry, breast milk is also a cure-all.

When Nicky was a month old, we traveled to Colorado, and the change in altitude made him congested and gave him his first stuffy nose. I was in a panic. I didn't know what to do for him, so I called my pediatrician. He said, "Get a small eyedropper, fill it with breast milk, and put drops of it in his nose." I couldn't believe it! Breast milk as a decongestant? But I was desperate, and sure enough, within seconds of inhaling a familiar taste, he was able to sleep through the night. The whole time I breast-fed, I was able to use breast milk for everything. Every time my boys had diaper rash or a cut or an allergic reaction to a new food, all I had to do was apply breast milk and the condition went away. Breast milk truly is one of God's miracles.

Breast-feeding Styles

All kids have their own style of breast-feeding. They say that kids can be classified in three categories: grazers, snackers, and feeders. Nicky was a feeder; Joey was a snacker. Nicky fed every four hours like clockwork, including the middle of the night. He finally slept through the morning at about five months old, unlike Joey, who snacked every two hours but would feed solidly before bedtime and slept through the night at three months old. You learn how each individual child feeds and you try to work it into your schedule. I am a big believer in on-demand feeding. That's how you learn your child's eating habits. You let them set it from the beginning. And gradually they will find their way into a schedule that eventually works for both of you.

It is important that your baby breast-feeds frequently throughout the day. This can be challenging when you are in public. Some women have no trouble doing it anytime, anywhere, while others are very modest. I was sort of in between. You will find that there is always someplace you can go—like department-store dressing rooms, bathrooms, or just in the corner somewhere. I found it really convenient to breast-feed, especially as a working mom who didn't want to bother with carrying a lot of cans and bottles.

Breast-feeding Tips

A good rule of thumb when breast-feeding is to keep a twelve-ounce tumbler of natural springwater next to you every time you breast-feed. It's important to replenish your fluids and this is a good way. Make sure you get ample amounts of protein during breast-feeding, too. Another great food to eat at this time is *mochi* (made from pounded brown rice). But mochi is not just good for breast-feeding moms. People talk about the benefits of mochi frequently on my Web site. It's incredible how many fans there are of mochi these days. Kids love mochi, too. They like to see it puff up. If you have never tried some, please do yourself the favor.

The first six weeks of breast-feeding establish the "rules." These weeks are amazing. You feel like Elsie the Cow. Your breasts are huge. Your body is still recovering from the delivery and you feel like a dairy farm because you are producing so much milk. It's actually a good time to pump; however, even though breast milk lasts a long time, I wouldn't overdo it. Remember that the breast milk you produce the first month is naturally formulated for your baby's first month of life. That's one of the incredible benefits of breast-feeding. Pumping and storing for three or four months minimizes this benefit. So even though breast milk can be kept two or three months in a regular open/close freezer and six months in a deep freezer, keep in mind that your baby is different at six weeks than she is at four months. Her nutritional needs are different, and what's great about your breast milk is that your baby's mouth communicates to your breast what kind of milk it should produce. The relationship can be so unbelievably pure and instinctual and natural if you just let nature take its course.

At first, you may be worried that you will run out of milk too soon. If you feed yourself well, you increase the odds that your body will continue to produce enough milk through the entire term. Many women start to panic because there tends to be less and less surplus as their baby grows. The reason is that you're feeding a child who is very small in the beginning, so you tend to have a surplus. But you can't store as much later on because your growing child demands more. At six weeks with Nicky, I thought, "What happened to my milk supply?" I started to feel really sad and fearful that I wasn't going to produce enough to feed him, especially since he was growing at a very rapid rate. Thankfully, everything worked out fine, perhaps because I did everything I could to put the odds in my favor: regular feedings, healthy diet, plenty of water, ample protein, mochi, and lots of green leafy vegetables. And I calmed down.

Here are some tips that have helped my friends and me while breast-feeding:

+ Breast-feeding should begin immediately after birth or as soon as possible. Make sure you have an understanding with your doctor and hospital.

+ Newborns nurse a lot. Ignore people who seem concerned that you are nursing too much. Breast milk is easily digested, so your baby may get hungry again after only an hour. This is normal. A baby should be fed at least eight to twelve times in twenty-four hours. Feed your baby every two to three hours. But remember that all babies are different. Some seem to nurse all the time and others go longer in between feedings.

+ Avoid bottles and pacifiers until breast-feeding is well established.

+ Make sure that the entire dark area around the nipple is in the baby's mouth. This will help stimulate milk flow and allow the baby to get enough milk. This will also prevent nipple soreness. Some babies have no trouble breast-feeding, while others need some assistance.

+ You'll learn a little bit more every day, so don't panic. Pain often means something is wrong with breast position in the baby's mouth. Don't simply endure it. Investigate what the problem might be and try to fix it. Talk to La Leche League. They can offer tons of help and support.

+ Air out your breasts as much as possible. After a feeding, don't immediately put them back in your bra. This helps prevent your nipples from getting overly sore and cracked.

+ You can tell if your baby is getting enough milk by checking her diapers. If she is wetting between four to six disposable diapers or six to eight cloth diapers and having two to three bowel movements in a twenty-four-hour period, she is getting enough.

+ Always dress comfortably and sit comfortably when you nurse. You could wind up with back trouble if you don't. Try resting your feet on a low stool, with knees raised slightly. Experiment with lots of pillows to find some comfortable positions, or invest in a nursing pillow to support your baby.

+ Set up contacts with friends and family who have a lot of experience with breast-feeding so you can turn to them for support when you need it.

+ You know the old expression "Use it or lose it"? This is true for breast-feeding, so nurse often.

+ Drink lots and lots of water. Drink while you are nursing.

Remember, there may be times when you and your baby will be frustrated, but many more times when you will both experience absolute joy.

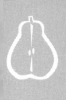

7

Infancy: Six Months to One Year

Introducing Solid Foods

Can you think of anything more exciting than feeding your baby something other than breast milk for the very first time? When Nicky turned six months old, Rob and I decided it was time for his first meal. We had gone to Toys "R" Us earlier that day and bought a new high chair, plastic-covered spoon, and bowl for the occasion. I prepared mashed bananas with a little bit of breast milk and Rob had the video camera ready and focused for this once-in-a-lifetime moment. I remember putting that first spoonful of banana in Nicky's mouth and watching his reaction. His head jerked back, his eyes opened wide, and his lips puckered. At first I thought he didn't like it, and then all of a sudden he opened his mouth and wanted more. I knew we had a match! Food was something he was ready for and banana was a taste sensation he really liked! It was what Nicky later called "my flavor." (To this day, when encouraged to try something new, Nicky asks, "Is that my flavor?")

Relatively speaking, he didn't really eat that much of the banana that day, but after six months of nothing but breast milk, he had entered a whole new world—the world of food! I knew it was only a matter of time before he'd be loading his plate at Beefsteak Charlie's. (I'm kidding!) I knew, from research, that you should introduce foods one at a time four days apart; this way you can make sure there are no allergic reactions. After feeding Nicky just a very small amount of banana every day for four days, I was looking forward to introducing his next food—a tiny bit of scraped pear, which I also mixed with breast milk. His reaction was the same as it had been with the banana; he loved it! He now had two foods in his gastronomic repertoire. I introduced new foods in this way every four or more days while I continued to breast-feed him. Breast milk was still his primary source of nutrition. This was a great way for him to get acquainted with new foods, see what he liked, and test for allergies. He seemed to enjoy and crave the same things I had craved when he was in the womb. Never having been much of a banana eater, I realized why I craved them so much during my pregnancy. Nicky must have been ordering them up like room service, or should I say "womb" service? I introduced Joey to the world of food the same way. Only he preferred melons.

During my pre- and postpregnancy research, I learned that one of the best ways to introduce food to your children is to let them play with it on their own. Let them experience the food, smell it, touch it, put it in their mouths, and develop their own independent relationship with it. The best way to feed a baby for the first time is to put a little bit of food on a plastic-covered baby spoon, place it near her mouth, and see if she'll take it in. Usually, she'll smell it, explore it, touch it with her tongue, and eventually put it in her mouth. She might spit it out; babies often do on the first try. If she does, try it again. If she spits it out after three tries, it's best to wait a few days before trying that particular food again. If babies want a food, you can usually tell. Their mouths will open and they'll eat it. I realized early on that it was important to feed my boys when they were hungry and stop feeding them when they weren't. This may sound obvious, but many parents force kids to eat or finish everything. This is a mistake. Knowing when a child wants more and when he doesn't is usually pretty clear. You'll see what I mean. An open mouth means "Yes, I want more." A closed mouth that pulls away means "I'm full, but please check back again at dinnertime."

Creating a Healthy Relationship with Food

Many parents have tight schedules and want their babies to get an ample amount of nutrition, so they often feed a child based on their own set plan and personal convenience, not the baby's. I see parents shovel food into their children's mouths at the same pace they feed themselves. An adult's pace is way too fast for a baby. It has more to do with finishing the jar than listening to the baby's needs. The best time to learn your child's natural hunger signals is during the first few feedings, before the child becomes influenced by the demands and pace set by the parent.

The more a parent can work with her child and understand the importance of this early stage of creating a healthy relationship with food, the bigger difference it will make later in the child's eating habits. As we have already discovered, the "clean plate syndrome" in adulthood can often be traced back to being forced to finish entire jars during that first year of baby food. One of the worst things a parent can say to a child at any age concerning diet is to finish everything on his plate. We adults are programmed to put a certain amount on our plate at each meal, and then we stop eating when our plate is empty, not when we're full. If you really pay attention to your child's hunger signals, you will see that he will eat very little at some meals and appear to be ravenous at others. This is why you should never predetermine the amount you are going to feed your baby at any meal. Watch for *their* signals.

I realized how important it was to let a child determine the timing of feeding when I watched a friend of mine feed her eight-month-old daughter while carrying on a very animated conversation with me. She and I were talking about something and she was all fired up while she was feeding her baby. I noticed that she was feeding her child faster and faster until it became almost comical because the baby couldn't get as much food in her mouth as my friend wanted to give her. My friend realized she had fed her baby the entire jar of baby food in a matter of about five minutes, and her daughter looked completely stuffed and ready to explode. I realized then how many times we all feed our children at the pace of an adult, and I made a vow never to feed my children without paying attention to when they wanted the next bite. Because of our adult schedule and need to get the job done, we parents often don't realize how quickly we feed our children, disregarding their natural appetite signals and pace.

Watching for Allergy Signs

I mentioned earlier that it is best to feed a child one food at a time, waiting four days before you introduce another food. By doing this, you can watch for any type of allergy signs—watery eyes, itchy nose, red ears, and so on. By introducing one food at a time and waiting four days, you will be able to notice any of the obvious reactions right after your child has eaten the new food. You will also be able to see if there is any reaction *after* your child has digested it, i.e., loose stool and/or diaper rash. Mix each food that you try with a little bit of your baby's usual fare (breast milk or formula). By doing this, you will not only minimize your baby's allergic reaction (if need be), but breast milk will also thin out the new food, which in its pure, whole state is at first too concentrated for his little system.

The following is a month-by-month guideline of how to introduce solid foods between the ages of six months to one year.

Food Introduction Guide

Age	Food
Birth through 18 months	Breast milk or soy-based, vitamin-enriched formula
6 to 7 months	Fruits: bananas, cooked peaches, cooked applesauce Later: raw, grated apple, pear, apricot, plums, melons, soaked fruit (Add liquid multivitamin/mineral supplement.)
7 to 8 months	Avocado, tofu, cooked green vegetables, mashed or blended carrots, yams, squash
10 months	Starchy foods: potatoes, whole grain cereals (oats, millet, rice, barley, etc.)
12 to 18 months (depending on baby's teeth)	Breads and pastas Cereals: rice, oats, wheat, etc. Legumes: peas, beans, chickpeas, lentils, soy products Nut butters: Almond, cashew, peanut

Ensuring Healthy and Safe Feeding Practices

You will notice that fruits are introduced first, followed by vegetables and tofu, followed by grains. So many people want to introduce grains to their child as a first food because they think it will make her sleep better, only to discover that their baby is up all night with a stomachache. There is nothing worse than feeding a child grains before she is ready to digest them, and one of the surest ways of knowing whether or not your child can digest grains is to check her teeth. If she doesn't have the teeth to indicate that she could "break" the grain, then she doesn't have the stomach enzymes needed to break it down. This doesn't mean she has to have molars, of course. She only has to have one or two teeth. If a child is having trouble teething, it usually means she is being fed something she can't handle, i.e., grains or protein.

One of the most important rules I learned when my children were this age was you should never let your baby fall asleep with a bottle. There is nothing worse for their teeth. It doesn't matter what's in the bottle, whether it's milk or formula or Rice Dream or juice, the natural sugars in those drinks will eventually cause problems with your child's teeth.

In very young children, the most important rule is to never put a child to sleep with a bottle that contains any sugary liquid. This would include milk, juice or soda. It causes rapid decay of teeth.—DR. MARK GOLDENBERG, D.D.S.

Another bit of advice that paid off was to never let my children walk around with a bottle. Walking around eating should not become a habit that starts at this age. It's also unsafe for children to have a bottle in their mouths while they are wandering around the house, especially at this age, when they are prone to falling.

8

· · · · · · · · · · ·

Toddler: Ages One to Two and a Half

I f there is one birthday that all parents remember celebrating, it is their child's first. The video camera is out, your baby is confidently sitting in his high chair, there are balloons everywhere, lots of presents, and it is usually your baby's first taste of birthday cake. I remember being excited to celebrate both of my boys' first birthdays because it was not only a rite of passage, it also marked the moment of their passing into an age at which I could feed them most of the foods that everyone else at the table was eating. Children at this age really seem to become part of the family's eating ritual since they can eat the same foods that you are eating, with exceptions of course. From six months to one year, my boys were eating mostly fruits, vegetables, tofu, and bread, pasta, and other easily mushed-up grains (because of course they did not have molars yet). But right after they turned one, I started giving them some fish and eggs (free-range, of course). Before one year of age you can give a child egg yolk and, after one, the whole egg. I remember being really excited about taking Nicky and Joey to a restaurant after each of their first birthdays because I knew I could order something right off the menu.

Creating an Independent Eater

A child starts to become an independent eater at this age, so the more you can encourage him to feed himself, the better off he will be. As I've explained throughout this book, it is the best way to teach a child how to have a relationship with food that honors his own sense of appetite and timing. Of course, at one year old, it is not possible for him to feed himself everything. But by two and a half, he should be able to do it all. However, at whatever age, make sure feeding himself is always done as safely as possible. Be sure to cut everything into pieces that are small enough to eliminate the risk of choking and be sure you keep a close eye on every bite and swallow. Letting a child feed himself is not an opportunity for a parent to make phone calls or watch TV. Make sure the pieces are not only bite-sized (*his* bite), but also that the temperature is not too hot or too cold. Check it out yourself first. Be prepared. Allowing your child to feed himself is, of course, going to be messy, but it is worth the mess if you want him to become an independent and natural eater. You should at least feed him this way at home as often as possible. A lot of food will end up on the high chair, the floor, your baby's hair, your hair, the dog's hair, everywhere. If you are worried about a mess, use a plastic drop cloth—a big one. Don't worry. The mess is worth it. This is the best way of all for a baby to develop his own relationship to food and his own appetite signals. And as always, give your child time to feed. Meals should take at least twenty minutes even when you are an adult, so why not start a nice healthy practice early on? Let your child realize that he is full by allowing him enough time to eat. He will tell you that he is full if he starts to play with his food. As soon as food becomes a plaything, the meal should be over.

Between one and two and a half years is the age when children explore their independence. I am now convinced that a lot of the terrible twos is exacerbated by an extreme diet. These little bodies do not know how to handle the chemicals and sugar in most of their food. Do not let mealtime become a battlefield. It is not worth it and it also sets up bad habits for later on.

Getting Them to "Chew"

I am always saying, "Your stomach doesn't have teeth." Learning how to chew food well is something few of us ever learn as children. Not only does chewing well help you get all of the vitamins and nutrients out of the food you eat, but it also prevents digestive problems. This is the perfect age to teach your child about chewing, but try to avoid white flour products with little nutritional value (teething biscuits, crackers, pretzels). Toast the heels of whole wheat bread or give raw carrot or apple to your older infant to practice chewing (or gumming). But in order to lower the risks of choking, never leave your child alone with food.

Establishing Good Social Habits

If you are the type of person who likes to dine in a restaurant with another family, one to two and a half years old is a great time in a child's life to introduce him to this experience. It is usually better not to let your kids get into the habit of running around with other kids in a restaurant where other people are trying to eat. If you let them get into this practice when they are this age, it is going to be extra hard to break them of it later on. Stick to noisy, family-friendly restaurants if you are with a lot of other kids, but try to make sure that the food you get is as healthy as possible. Otherwise, within fifteen minutes of their eating sugary and/or salty overprocessed food, you are going to have children who are impossible to control. If your children have not been eating extreme foods, chances are they will sit nicely or at least nicely enough for you to get about forty-five minutes (or maybe even an hour!) of decent dining time. Winning those little battles of good behavior at this age will pay off in the long run. In other words, the more positive habits you establish now, the fewer bad habits you will have to break later on.

Two days before we started THM we went out with some friends. It was about seven or eight P.M. and the kids were all sitting nicely together—one six-year-old, one five-year-old, two four-year-olds, and a three-year-old. My husband bought my kids some cookies (with sugar and dairy) and the other mother bought her children some brownies (also with sugar and *dairy). In about ten minutes we heard and saw that my four-year-old was on the ground and the other children including my oldest child were standing around. Upon closer inspection I realized that these young children, all friends with each other, were pretty much KICKING MY SON IN THE STOMACH. We separated them and they were screaming and causing such a fuss that I took them outside to play. Fast-forward nine months: our family is now THMers and the meltdowns that I thought were a part of life NO LONGER EXIST. If my children do cry, it is for only a minute or two and then it's okay. I am so glad that meltdowns are no longer normal behavior for my children!—*SLEEKER, MARILU.COM

Sharing food is a great social event, so the more you can expose your child to sharing a meal with other people, the better off you and they will be. Your child will be curious about other people's food, and of course she will want to try what is on someone else's plate. If you let her do that, make sure that the food contains nothing that your child might be allergic to or have a reaction to. And also make sure it is not too hot, too cold, or too spicy.

Transitioning from Unhealthy to Healthy Foods

If your child has been snacking on Cheerios and soda pop (or high-fructose corn-syrup-sweetened fruit juices), you may want to wean him away from those extreme foods, and it is easy to do at this age. There are so many wonderful products in health food stores. For example, Oatios is superior to Cheerios; not only is it made from whole grains, it does not contain refined sugar or chemicals. I see so many children walking around with little baggies of Cheerios and Goldfish, and I always want to ask their parents if they have read the label. There are many other cereals and snack foods that you can find in a health food store that are not too sweet or too salty. At this age we have the golden opportunity to create a healthy palate, one that is sensitive to subtle flavors and not one that will only desire extreme salt and extreme sugar. So why not do what is best for our children in the long run?

Carbonated soda pop provides more added sugar in a typical two-year-old toddler's diet than cookies, candy, and ice cream combined.

Washington Post,
February 27, 2001

In my daughter's kindergarten class (public school), each child brings in their own drink each day (juice box, water bottle, etc.) and they take turns bringing in a big box or bag of snack food so everyone is eating the same thing every day. My daughter is the only one to bring in her own snack. The other kids are always interested in what she has. One day she brought in some Veggie Booty and blew everybody away!—MARILU.COM, USER

If you have been giving your child soft drinks, especially the ones with caffeine, it would be better to switch to 100 percent fruit juice (without high-fructose corn syrup) watered down by a half to two-thirds with natural springwater. (Or Original Enriched Rice Dream, Soy Dream, or other nondairy healthy drinks if you have decided to take my advice and raise your child in a nondairy way.) I cannot tell you the number of times I have seen children in a stroller with a can of Coke or Diet Coke or Hawaiian Punch, only to see them crying or whining minutes later.

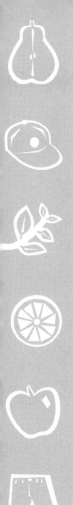

9

Preschool: Ages Two and a Half to Five

And they're off!

There is no time in a child's life when she has more energy than at two and a half to five years old. Your toddler turns into a real person, and you can't believe it. It seems like only yesterday that they were holding a bottle, and now they're handing you a drawing for the refrigerator. The world is an exciting place indeed for a child who can move around and discover all of it, including the world of food.

Setting up a healthy kitchen at home is now more important than ever because a child this age is taking what she learns at home into the outside world. If you can introduce your child to a variety of foods, this is the time to do it. Her palate is developing, and by the time she is five, she will know exactly what she likes, no *if*s, *and*s, or *but*s. That's why if you can get in there and introduce her to healthy food before five, you won't have as much "undoing" to do later.

My four-year-old daughter loves broccoli, but her mother taught her to eat it drenched in butter. When she asked me to butter her broccoli when she was eating with me on the weekends, I refused. She didn't like it at first, but agreed to eat it anyway. Once she got about two or three bites into it, she forgot all about the butter and enjoyed her broccoli. Once her mom got on board with me, we were able to train our daughter's palate in a healthy way.—WILLIE WILSON, GEORGIA

Preschool and Play Dates

Your child will be starting preschool during this time, and with it comes a whole new world. Not only will he be eating food away from home provided by another source, but he will be introduced to the social swirl of play dates, birthday parties, and other families' food agendas (unwittingly or not!). The best thing to do at school is to talk to your child's teacher or the head of the school and let them know in writing what your child can or cannot eat. With my sons, I listed sugar, meat, and dairy. Schools want to know this information and they will usually work with you. Believe me, no school wants to deal with the consequences of your child reacting to something on the list. Try to find the teacher who is most sympathetic to your cause. (Who knows, there may be a THM convert on staff!) You may want to explain to them that your child is allergic to dairy (because she's not a baby calf). My son Nicky has a runny nose for three days if he inadvertently (or purposely) eats something with dairy in it.

When your child is going on a play date, call ahead to the mom and tell her what is on your family's forbidden list. There is usually something in someone else's pantry and refrigerator that your child can eat. You just need to discuss it ahead of time. No one wants to entertain a child in their home and not have him eat something, so if you are not sure your child will eat what other people have, you can always pack something for him to take along. My kids will eat fruit, or pasta with tomato sauce, or peanut butter and jelly. Let's put it this way. Whatever your kids eat someplace else, even if it's bad for them, can be made up for later at home. You want your kids to be able to live in the outside world, so you might have to relax the rules a little until the world catches up. But at this age it is easier to set up the rules and communicate them to your child's teacher and play date parents.

Your Child's Eating Habits and Others

Grandparents are a whole other matter! They seem to love indulging their grandkids with lots of tantalizing sweets and other junk food. I think they are in denial that these treats are, in fact, junk food because they are similar to what they fed us when we were kids. They didn't know any better. When we try to discourage them, they'll say things like "Come on. You ate that when you were a kid and you turned out okay." I always explain to people that for all the junk we ate as kids, we were still eating more real food than any of our kids eat today. And our parents and our grandparents ate more real food than we did. It's more important than ever to get your parents on board and take some responsibility for their grandkids' nutrition. But even if you can't get through to your parents, remember that you can always undo what they've done. Don't let food turn into a battle. You are better off changing your family's palate slowly but surely so that they don't even want the unhealthy foods anymore.

We went to a birthday party last Saturday at McDonald's and took our own soy burgers. I also took juice boxes and water for me. The kids ate some French fries but didn't go nuts over them like I thought they would. The mother of the kid having the party knew we would do this, as I had spoken to her days in advance. Still, she made two comments to me, in a teasing way, that I was a mean mother. I responded that if she saw it from my point of view, she would understand, and if my son were a diabetic, it wouldn't be an issue. She agreed. Now, I am not in a position to tell others what to do about their kids, but I am in control of mine. I let my son have a small piece of cake, but he barely ate it.—SUZANNE "SUZALL" PALUMBO, GEORGIA

A child's eating habits at age 3 can help predict whether or not he or she will have a mouthful of cavities by the time they are age 6. Toddlers who consumed candy and juice more than once a week at age 3 and who also had tartar-bacteria-containing plaque on the teeth were nearly twice as likely to have cavities by the age of 6, compared with their peers who ate sweets no more than once a week, findings show.

Dentistry and Oral Epidemiology, 2001

Another rite of passage during this time is your child's first trip to the dentist, usually around two and a half to three years old. If you find out that your child

139

has soft teeth and is on her way to developing cavities, it is crucial that you change your family's health habits now.

List of Favorite Fruits and Vegetables

Children 2½ to 5

Favorite Fruits	*Favorite Vegetables*
1. Apple	1. Carrots
2. Watermelon	2. Broccoli
3. Banana	3. Cucumbers
4. Grapes	4. Lettuce
5. Cantaloupe	5. Spinach
6. Strawberries	6. String beans
7. Pears	7. Celery
8. Oranges	8. Corn
9. Cherries	9. Peas
10. Peaches	10. Cabbage

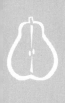

10
· · · · · · · · · · ·

Elementary School:
Ages Six to Nine

Six to nine years old can be a great age to get your child healthy. Not only are they at an age where they can understand the connection between food and health (as in what they eat and how it makes them feel), but children tend to be natural vegetarians at this age. If you are thinking about exploring vegetarianism for your whole family, this may be a good time to start. In fact, many children at this age choose to become vegetarian on their own because they usually make the connection between killing animals and eating them. They become socially conscious and begin to understand how animals are killed for food. They start to realize that the beef you are serving was once a cow and that the chicken leg was once, well . . . exactly that. Many people on my Web site or friends of mine have told me that their whole family is becoming interested in health because their child (who is usually in this age group) now refuses to eat anything "with a face."

Profile of a Consumer

They call seven the age of reason, but eight years old really seems to be the age when children need to be able to reason the most, because this age seems to be most targeted by Madison Avenue, from fast food to music. Eight seems to be the age most industries consider crucial; if they get you as a consumer then, they have you for life. If they start to target at three, they will have a certified customer by the time a child is eight.

It is interesting to note that most teachers, PE teachers, and doctors whom I talked to said that by eight years old a child becomes rather set in his ways. When I interviewed Susan Cole, the PE teacher at my sons' school, she said that by the time a child is eight, he is pretty much the athlete he is going to be. Before eight, you can get the child to jump around the playground and play games, but often at this age, a child has decided whether or not he has a propensity for sports. According to Susan Cole, there is a self-consciousness that tends to take over around this age. Kids tend to see the world as all or nothing. She claims that at this age kids either start to get sluggish or they decide they are an athlete and really into sports. The sluggish ones start to put on weight and become less alert. She sees it mostly in boys. If they're not the superstars, if they're not totally into sports, they tend to withdraw from PE class activities. The girls, on the other hand, start becoming conscious of their weight, and this is where, in her experience, she sees eating disorders take hold. She sees a lot of girls around this age refuse to eat and feel the pressure to be pretty and thin. Dr. Peter Waldstein agrees. "I see these kids and their bodies are getting mature but their minds are not, so it's hard to handle. They want to be thin because all they see on television are pop stars with tight little stomachs, and these kids want to emulate them. Well, how do they emulate them? They don't exercise, they stop eating, and they get themselves into an eating disorder."

This is also the age when kids start to get junk food on their own, especially from vending machines and snack bars. They are not eating what their parents want them to eat, and they open themselves to eating

A study by Texas A&M University showed that children develop brand loyalty at a very early age. Young people independently spend more than $2 billion a year on food, and influence $75 billion of the total amount spent on foods by adults.

Smart Medicine for a Healthy Child

junk food with their friends. This is why it is so important to teach this age group about healthy eating habits, to make them conscious of how the world is targeting them from all areas, and to show them how to discern the bad from the good. Just as the fast food industry and the music industry believe they will have a consumer for life by advertising, so you will have a healthy child for life if you can help them make the connection between what they eat and how they feel. The trick is to get them to help you help them.

Getting Them to Pack Their School Lunch

Kids six to nine are naturally curious and naturally helpful. One of the things I especially recommend at this age when they want to be independent is that you get them involved with packing their own lunch. You can do it at a younger age, of course, but six to nine is the time when you will most want their input so that the food gets eaten. One of my friend's pediatricians, when asked, "What should I pack for my child's lunch?" replied, "Whatever you want to eat in the car when you pick him up from school." The best way to avoid your getting an extra meal at 3:15 is to take your kids shopping (at a health food store whenever possible) and have them pick out the foods that you mutually agree on. Kids follow by example, so (hopefully) they will at least *try* to put something healthy in their lunch boxes because they have seen you do it so many times. Get them to pack their lunch so that they feel involved in what they have chosen and are therefore going to eat it. I ran an experiment with my boys this past year in which I had them help me pack their own lunches. It was amazing to me how much more often they ate their lunches because they felt invested in what they put together.

If you've never shopped in a health food store, you may want to let your child experiment with dif-

University of Michigan's Kristen Harrison, Ph.D., an assistant professor of communication studies, surveyed 300 children ages six through eight about their television viewing habits, character preferences, and perceptions about ideal body type. Using the Children's Eating Attitude Test—a battery of questions targeting restrained eating aimed at weight loss—Harrison found that as the kids' overall TV viewing hours increased per week, so did their number of disordered eating symptoms.

Psychology Today, 1999

ferent foods at first. You might make a few mistakes and you might buy some things you don't like, but buying what your child is attracted to on the shelf is a great way to introduce her to healthy foods. The health food industry has finally caught up with the processed food industry in making their packaging more colorful and attractive to children.

Take the kids with you to the health food store. It really does help if they can choose things themselves.—MARY BETH BORKOWSKI, NEW JERSEY

Change the eating habits slowly so healthy eating becomes a habit, and allow the kids to have input about their meals. You might choose the bread and the brand of peanut butter, but they can pick the flavor of jelly, or whether to have apple or pear slices. At dinner, I always let my kids decide on their vegetable, even if it's different from what I'm having.
—VALERIE DURBIN, CALIFORNIA

It is also easier to get children to make the connection between what they eat and how they feel at this age, especially if they are involved in any kind of sports.

Good nutrition is of course important at any age, but it's really important at this growing time in a child's life. People who are educated in good nutrition will provide it for their children, and those who lack the knowledge and the resources will not.—JOHN FISCHER, COFOUNDER HOOPMASTERS, YOUTH BASKETBALL PROGRAM, LOS ANGELES, CALIFORNIA

This is worth noting because after reading this book you can't choose not to know anymore. What I am trying to do is explain to you why it is so important for your child to eat healthy foods, and I hope enough of this knowledge will sink in so that you can teach your child how to do it for himself.

Dead Food at Lunch, Dead Tired All Day!

As school gets more difficult and the pressure to succeed starts to mount, it is even more important to teach children proper nutrition. Classes get harder and tests are more frequent. More homework needs to be done in the evening, and this requires a more sustained, consistent supply of energy and sense of well-being throughout the day. These can only be achieved by fueling the body with healthy food. Adding to the pressure are the ERB or standardized tests, which start in the third grade. Every child I know is in a panic during this time because he is old enough to know what these test scores mean to the rest of the school. It is very important that your child feels ready to handle the natural anxiety these tests cause. The best way to do this is to make sure they have not eaten extreme foods the day before or the morning of. They should not be eating extreme foods anyway, but especially during that test-taking period when stress can take its toll, especially on a body that's already stressed from the wrong kinds of food.

Being a room mother at one time, I noticed how many children would eat dead food at lunch and then feel dead tired all afternoon. As I have already suggested, the best way to get your children to eat a healthy lunch is to have them pack it. But regardless of who packs it, kids are going to trade their lunches. The best thing you can do is find out what they are trading and why they are trading it. Armed with this information, take them to the health food store and find the healthy versions. Everything is available nowadays. Years ago there was nothing and now there is a wonderful marriage between health foods and convenience foods. Sometimes children trade not because of the food itself but because of its packaging. Now you can compete with that portable chemistry set (aka Lunchables) by creating your own nicely packaged healthy lunch. All you have to do is find plastic containers with compartments and fill them with healthy versions of the foods your child is most likely to trade for. Find interesting ways to present the food as well. Use a cookie cutter to shape toasted sandwiches or provide a small container of dressing with cut up vegetables. It's amazing how much more often your kid will eat a tuna sandwich shaped like a star.

Last year one of my daughter's favorite lunches was a Mexican cream cheese dip. You know the one you always get at parties in the summer? I took a flat plastic container and spread soy cream cheese on the bottom. Top with salsa, fresh tomatoes and cucumbers (chopped), shredded lettuce, soy cheddar, olives, onions, whatever veggies your kids like. Send some Bearitos corn chips along with some carrot and celery sticks for dipping, zucchini sticks, cucumber slices—whatever!—MARY BETH BORKOWSKI, NEW JERSEY

Here are more lunch box snack suggestions:

Lunch Box Snacks

1. Veggie sticks (carrots, celery, zucchini, cucumbers)
2. Fresh fruit cubes (oranges, pineapple, apple slices rubbed with lemon, melons, bag of grapes) or make into fruit kabobs
3. Popcorn
4. Pretzels
5. Nuts
6. Trail mix
7. Celery with raisins and peanut butter on top
8. Soy yogurt topped with fresh fruit in a thermos
9. Soy cheese and crackers
10. Graham crackers
11. Dried fruits (mangos, papaya, pineapples)
12. Tortilla chips with salsa in a cup
13. Soup in a thermos
14. Pickles
15. Hard-boiled eggs

Children at this age will start to develop a sense of pride in eating this way if you do. If you can get your child to explain to you his understanding of why your family eats the way it does now, you will be amazed at how much he has learned. Solicit his help in explaining it to one of your friends or his or to a younger sibling. So much depends on your attitude. If you make a game out of finding or creating the healthy version of the foods you used to eat, it can be a lot of fun for both of you.

If you throw a sleepover at your house, go to the health food store and get chips and popcorn and everything else the kids are used to eating, but put it in bowls. They won't know the difference if they don't see the bags they are used to seeing. I am telling you, because of the availability of great food, it is not difficult to become a healthy family. I have seen people change their entire family around because they were so committed to doing so. It may take a while, but as I said before, it is worth the effort. You will almost immediately notice a change in your children's behavior when they eat more centered foods or more centered versions of the foods they are used to eating. But you have to be committed. You have to start doing little things like having a big bowl of fresh cut-up vegetables and fruits for them when they come home from school. If something healthy is available and ready to eat when they are hungry, they will grab it. Another thing you may want to experiment with is feeding your children their dinner right after school, when they are most ravenous. This will ensure that they eat something healthy rather than snacking on something bad for them. You can always feed them something lighter at dinnertime. Over time, as they wean themselves off extreme food, they will calm down and sit with you at dinnertime.

List of Favorite Fruits and Vegetables

Children 6 to 9

Favorite Fruits	*Favorite Vegetables*
1. Apple	1. Carrots
2. Grapes	2. Broccoli
3. Oranges	3. Potato
4. Watermelon	4. Lettuce
5. Banana	5. Peas
6. Strawberries	6. Cucumber
7. Peach	7. Celery
8. Pears	8. Cauliflower
9. Pineapple	9. Peppers
10. Cantaloupe	10. Green beans

11

. . . .

Adolescence: Ages
Ten to Thirteen

According to a new study, 9- to 14-year-old children who dine with their parents tend to have healthier diets—they consume less fried foods and more fruit and vegetables and essential nutrients—than those who don't.

Parenting, September 2000

Adolescence—yikes!

A child is caught in that world between trying to stay a child and trying to act like a grown-up. She doesn't know whether to sit on your lap or slam the door. As parents, we want to hang on to our little girl or boy, but we know that they are ready to move on. It is a difficult transition for both parent and child, made even more difficult by poor nutrition. That is why good health and eating habits are more important than ever. Your child is not only becoming more of a social creature and more interested in the world outside her family circle, but her body is changing so rapidly that many times the body is ready but the mind is not.

Raging Hormones

If there is ever a time for a child to eat centered foods as often as possible, it is during adolescence. As we already know, extreme food creates extreme behavior, and if your adolescent is riding the Raging Hormone (aka the emotional roller coaster), eating only extreme salt and extreme sugar, no way is she going to enjoy the ride of her life. Children at this age are extremely sensitive and have a tendency to feel that the world, and especially their parents, is against them. They think everyone is prettier than they are or a better athlete, and they are reactive to everything you say and do.

In the past few years, we have seen the onset of menstruation go from twelve to around ten years old, according to Dr. Peter Waldstein. This was unheard of when I was a kid. Most girls got their periods around twelve, thirteen, or even fourteen. But the age has lowered, and many studies point to the hormones in our food. Think about it. If we are pumping enough hormones into our cows and chickens to get them to produce up to fifteen times more than they naturally would, what do you think it's doing to our children's bodies?

As far as biggest health problems our kids are facing, I would say the antibiotics, hormones, etc., put into the animals that the kids end up ingesting (my daughter started her period at age nine, and I truly believe it's related to what we are eating).—MARILU.COM USER, MINNESOTA

Connection Between Dairy and Bad Skin

The dramas of puberty very often include the drama of bad skin. I remember when my stepson Lorne came to live with his father and me. He was thirteen at the time and was seeing an allergy doctor for his acne. Every two weeks he would get shots. He took allergy medication, and he walked around with an inhaler. He was also putting keto sticks in his urine every morning to test his pH levels. I took a good look at his skin, and because I was able to observe his daily eating habits, I recognized that most of what he ate contained dairy products. After a few days, I called his allergist and said, "Lorne may be allergic to some of the pollens you told him about, but I think he has more of a problem with dairy." The doctor said, "Oh no, no, no. Bad skin has nothing to do with what you eat." "Okay, thank you," I said, but I knew I had to take matters into my own hands. I made a wager with Lorne, betting him that he couldn't give up dairy for the six weeks while I went away on a job that summer. He was reluctant to take me up on my wager but finally agreed because I told him it only had to be for six weeks. Six weeks later I could not believe the difference. He had stopped sniffling, he didn't need his shots anymore, he didn't need his allergy medication, and he didn't need his inhaler. I saw a completely different boy. His body changed, he stopped looking doughy, and most important to him, his skin got better. It was as if a miracle had taken place, but all it involved was getting rid of dairy.

If your child has any of the problems that I have mentioned throughout this book—stuffy nose, ear infections, sore throats, bed-wetting, digestion problems or stomachaches, bad skin, or significant weight gain—especially during this sensitive age, I urge you to take her off dairy products for three weeks to a month to see if any of these conditions improves. I am sure the results will be enough to inspire you to keep her off dairy—permanently.

Many times you can get your children to eat healthier if you are consistent with your own health habits or if they observe the reaction to bad food in other people. You have to educate them and then trust that they will make the connection. But remember, they will never make the connection unless you are diligent about educating them all of the time.

After a year my kids are realizing that this is not one of Mom's phases. They are seeing the benefits of eating this way. Some of my eleven-year-old son's best friends are overweight, and he sees that they never eat veggies and they drink pop with everything. He gets frustrated when they can't keep up with him physically and just want to sit around playing video games. I have told him the way they eat steals their energy. He believes it now. My thirteen-year-old daughter saw her friends change a lot the first year of junior high. Their skin breaks out; they're getting a little chubby. I asked her why she thought this was happening to them and she said they all have fries and Dr Pepper for lunch. In track she ran the mile and noticed that when she did not eat a good lunch, she could not run. When she ate well, she was a LOT faster.—GERI, ARIZONA

And sometimes the connection takes a while but happens nonetheless.

I was an overweight child growing up. In seventh grade they called me "thunder thighs." In high school, I never had a date. I can tell you right now, that is something you never leave completely behind you. It wasn't until I read Total Health Makeover *two years ago that I had any clue what was in the Mac & cheese, Hamburger Helper, and Twinkies.*

—RENÉE, CALIFORNIA

List of Favorite Fruits and Vegetables

Children 10 to 13

Favorite Fruits	*Favorite Vegetables*
1. Apple	1. Carrots
2. Oranges	2. Broccoli
3. Strawberries	3. Celery
4. Banana	4. Lettuce
5. Grapes	5. Potato
6. Pineapple	6. Corn
7. Watermelon	7. Tomato
8. Peach	8. Cucumber
9. Pear	9. Green beans
10. Kiwi	10. Peas

12

Teenagers: Ages Fourteen to Eighteen

I t was the best of times, it was the worst of times.

Can you remember a time that was more yin and yang than high school? I can to this day remember feeling my absolute best and my absolute worst . . . all within an hour! In the four short years of high school, you go from being the awkward, insecure freshman to being the big-shot, know-it-all senior. And everything in between!

A Time of Emotional Extremes

The teenagers I interviewed for this book convinced me more than ever that it's not like it was when we were kids. The questions are the same: "Where do I fit in?" "Do people like me?" "How do I compare to everyone else?" "Will that boy ask me out?" "Will that girl say no if I ask her out?" But it is more complicated than this because the pressures of the world have shifted dramatically. The world is so much bigger now and, at the same time, more available, thanks to modern technology. It's almost impossible to control your teenager today, but the thing you can do more than anything else is to set a consistently good example. Even if most of your teenager's meals are eaten away from the house, if you eat well and set up a healthy kitchen at home, you will be surprised and amazed at how much she sounds like you when she gets together with her friends.

The biggest problem with feeding teenagers at school is that they have absolutely no time to sit down and eat anything decent for lunch. They have so little time to socialize with their friends since the school gives them only about thirty minutes to eat. So everything is done on the run. The tendency is to grab a candy bar and a soda at the vending machines. I really believe that vending machines at school and the fast food industry have been the major contributors to the downfall of good health and nutrition in kids. Teenagers want the quick fill at lunch, so they grab a bag of salty chips and/or a sugary candy bar and wash it down with a soda. Most of them don't eat breakfast unless they grab a white flour bagel or a sugar-heavy granola bar, but more often than not, their first meal is at eleven o'clock. And what is their food for the rest of the day? Mostly junk. The white foods—white flour, white sugar, dairy, processed food. Nothing with any nutritional value, only food that keeps them amped up and a little crazy all day long.

And the exercise situation at school is worse. Usually there is a daily gym class, but it's only about thirty or forty minutes long. Kids don't take showers at school anymore (unless they're involved in after-school sports), so the gym class isn't active enough for them to sweat. And very few of them do any other form of physical activity throughout the week.

Junk Food, Acne, Pride, and Vanity

What is also amazing to me is that so many teenagers are self-conscious enough about their skin to endure trips to the dermatologist, who gives them medication, shots, creams, ointments, and various treatments to improve it, but they still eat junk. If they took care of their skin from the inside out, it would make such a difference, not only in how they look but also how they feel.

Teenagers know what to do to be healthier, they just don't want to think about it. They know they should be drinking less soda and eating fewer fast foods, but they think, "Who cares? I'm young. I'll deal with that later."

The best way to make inroads with teenagers is to appeal to their sense of vanity. Try to talk to them about food and its connection to their skin, their weight, their muscle tone, and their energy. Talk to them or give them something to read. The situation doesn't have to be hopeless. They want to rebel against you, but it's better if they don't rebel against themselves at the same time. Most teenagers live in the world of "I'll show you," doing whatever it is that you *don't* want them to do. But they are really hurting themselves in the long run. If you are having problems with your teenager's health habits, perhaps you can appeal to a person that he admires. You may be able to solicit that person's help in convincing your teenager to eat better. You may have to do it slowly but surely, but if you can turn him on to the world of health, I promise you he will thank you for it later.

My son grudgingly gave up the dairy when his normal complexion erupted unmercifully. I don't think health meant a thing to him. His girlfriend meant a lot, though. Dermatology treatments were ineffective when he cheated with the dairy. I can see it in his face right away when he isn't diligent. He also has always had back-to-back colds from the fall to the spring until this year. He has terrible allergies and a deviated septum, and has had to miss school in past years because he was miserable. He just said to me the other night, "Mom, I haven't been sick or had even one cold all year. You were right!" I love hearing that from my kids.—Mary Beth Borkowski, New Jersey

My son is eighteen and my daughter is fourteen and we have been eating healthy for a year and a half. They are, on their own, choosing to eat this way when they are out with their friends. They are really enjoying the flavor of the food they eat now. When the garbage is out of their system, teenagers will enjoy good fresh food. My daughter is a dancer. I think this prevents the tendency, at this age, to focus on her weight, which can be dangerous. Instead, the emphasis is on how well she feels, how much energy she has. I love this because it helps them to enjoy their lives, get more out of each day, and be the best version of themselves that they can be.

—Mary Beth Borkowski, New Jersey

How to Deal with Cigarette Smoking

It is also difficult for teenagers to make the connection between smoking and cancer. When you are fourteen, dying at sixty-five instead of seventy-five doesn't seem like a big deal. But the threat of looking forty-five when you're really thirty-five might. Researches in the U.K. recently found a connection between smoking and premature aging. Tobacco contains chemicals that have a damaging effect on the skin and cause it to look older than it actually is. Tobacco smoke triggers an increase in the protein matrix metalloproteinase 1 (MMP-1), which breaks down collagen and causes a breakdown in the elasticity of the skin. Doctors at Guy's, King's, and St. Thomas's schools of medicine in London were studying the effects of ultraviolet light on skin when they realized smokers have high levels of the same protein found in people who have had excessive exposure to the sun. Antony Young, a photobiology professor, and his team aren't sure which of the thousands of chemicals in tobacco activate the gene, but they suspect it's the same as those that cause cancer because MMP-1 also has been linked to the disease.

My son Joey has the best take on smoking I have ever heard. One day he said to me, "I think grown-ups think smoking is a magic trick." I said, "What do you mean, a magic trick?" He said, "They think you can put poison in your body and it won't hurt you."

And he's five years old.

> Teenagers who smoked at least 20 cigarettes a day had 12 times the risk of suffering panic attacks and 5 times the risk of generalized anxiety disorder and agoraphobia.
>
> *New York Times,*
> *November 8, 2000*

List of Favorite Fruits and Vegetables

Teenagers 14 to 18

Favorite Fruits

1. Apple
2. Banana
3. Orange
4. Grapes
5. Pineapple
6. Peaches
7. Strawberries
8. Cantaloupe
9. Grapefruit
10. Cherries

Favorite Vegetables

1. Carrots
2. Broccoli
3. Cauliflower
4. Peas
5. Green beans
6. Corn
7. Lettuce
8. Tomato
9. Potato
10. Spinach

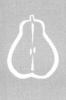

13

College: Eighteen Plus

One of the most exciting but stressful times in the life of a child (or a parent!) is going off to college. She asks herself, "Where am I going to live?" "What is the neighborhood like?" "Will I have a nice roommate?" "Will I make the dean's list?" But most of all she wonders, "Will I gain the freshman fifteen?" The freshman fifteen is that dreaded fifteen pounds that almost everyone puts on their first year of college. I not only gained the freshman fifteen, I was so anxious to get to college that I gained an additional twenty-five the summer before I even got there. It happens because not only are you away from home for the first time dealing with the stress of independence, but you are also dealing with the joy of being able to eat as much as you want whenever you want. The only problem is that you are dependent on what kind of food they serve at your dorm. Most people choose to live in a dorm their first year in order to adjust to college life, and even though it can be one of the happiest times for socializing and getting to know the people in their class, it is also conducive to bad eating habits. There are any number of reasons for this, the most obvious being the quality of food they usually serve in dorms. After doing extensive research on the subject, I have discovered that, yes, dorm food has gotten better since I went to college, but not by that much. There are, however, certain things that you can do to avoid gaining the famous freshman fifteen.

Avoiding the Freshman Fifteen

First of all, I would recommend that freshmen don't do what most college kids do their first year, which is to add drinking beer and eating pizza to their weekend. Two slices of cheese pizza and two beers twice a week adds an additional 63,633 mindless calories per school year. (And who are we kidding when we say we're going to have only two beers!) That's an additional eighteen pounds per year. Each weekend adds an extra thousand mindless calories if you don't change anything else about your diet. This is the guaranteed way of gaining the freshman fifteen or more. The key word here is *mindless*, because eating should never be mindless. If you must order pizza, follow the food-combining rules and order it with mushrooms, olives, sun-dried tomatoes (or any other vegetables), but no cheese! College is the time when you train your mind. You can begin with your diet. Mind what you eat.

When I think about my college experience, I realize if I had known then what I know now I probably could have treated it like a spa instead of a Las Vegas buffet—anything and everything at all hours of the day and night. While food was available in all forms, both healthy and unhealthy, now that I know how to eat anywhere and stay on the program, I could have been clever in avoiding the bad foods and relishing the good ones. The important thing to do is to go to your dorm cafeteria and size up what is available to you. Most of the schools have an all-you-can-eat salad bar, which means you can load up on fresh vegetables and fruits. If they only offer you dressings full of chemicals or dairy products or fat-free but full of chemicals, you are better off investing in your own salad dressing—for example, Annie's or Paul Newman's. Pick a brand that will add flavor without adding chemistry. Or if you really want to be fancy, get some virgin olive oil and balsamic vinegar. You can use my salad bag trick, which is to get a large plastic bag, put your salad in it, pour in a capful of dressing, blow some air into the bag, and shake it up. You will have a well-dressed salad with very few calories and very little fat.

You might also want to look into food-combining because most college dorms serve three meals a day, so you will be eating enough throughout the day. If you are the typical college student you will be hungry all the time, so you might as well food-combine. It is unlikely that you will gain weight if you do, especially if you pay attention to portions. (Please see food-combining chart on page 302–303.) And stay away from all the white foods as much as possible—white sugar, white processed flour, and dairy products. As I have explained throughout this book, the white foods will take energy from you rather than give you the energy you need to face all of your academic responsibilities.

Making Dorm Food Healthier

College is really an exciting time in a person's life, so you don't want to lose the social aspect of eating in the dorm with your friends. But that doesn't mean you have to pig out or eat all of the unhealthy foods you find in dorms. What is great about dorms today is that most of them offer a vegetarian entrée, a vegan entrée, a low-fat entrée (under 30 percent), and a meat entrée. If none of them look appealing that day, you may want to check out the side dishes and jazz them up with something you bring from the outside that will add some flavor and some nutrients. My advice would be to get a spray bottle of Bragg Liquid Aminos, which is very tasty and full of amino acids. Once you get into the flavor, you will end up putting it on everything from vegetables to eggs to fish to air-popped popcorn.

Another way to make sure that you are getting your vitamins and minerals is to buy a package of seaweed nori. This is the seaweed that is used when making sushi, and is one of the most convenient, nutrient-dense foods you can buy. You can make your own wraps using the various foods from the salad bar. You will be making an entrée out of your salad-bar food and you are sure to get all of the vitamins and minerals that you need.

Freshness is often a problem in dorms because the food has been sitting around or it is not of the same quality as you would find in a good grocery store or health food store. The produce is not going to be organic, so it is necessary to supplement it with vitamins as much as possible. And on those occasions when you've seen a version of the same entrée for the third night in a row, you may want to buy something to supplement your dinner. Become familiar with your local health food store, and once in a while you can buy a ready-made entrée that you can pop in the microwave. Health food has become extremely convenient in the past five years and plenty of inexpensive microwavable food is available. You don't have to be a gourmet chef to create a healthy meal when dorm food is not enough.

My son is a college sophomore. He eats a very healthy diet. He was never very happy with the university food service. He manages to eat well by taking extra fruit from the cafeteria for a morning snack. He keeps soup cups and oatmeal in his room. I also send him Uncle Eddie's Vegan cookies on occasion.—EDNA AXELROD, NEW JERSEY

It was interesting to note that among the college students I polled, those who gained the freshman fifteen said that their diets consisted mostly of the white foods. They were more likely to add cheese to their salads or drank milk a lot throughout the day. Dairy products, especially coupled with the other white foods, sugar and white flour, really pack on the weight, especially in an environment where you tend to do a lot of mindless eating while studying. (What a concept!) What was interesting to note in the surveys was that among the students who ate oatmeal for breakfast (and there were many of them who chose oatmeal as a breakfast staple), not *one* of them put on the freshman fifteen. The conclusion I draw from that is if you start your day with a whole grain cereal full of fiber, even if you are not eating well the rest of the day, you will be getting rid of all of it at some point and it won't hang around in there.

Whatever the situation at your dorm, you can always improve it by getting involved. It is easy to sit back and complain, but to be really effective in raising the quality of the food you eat, you should get involved and talk to the people in charge or fill out comment cards or meet with the food committee. Even though you are a college student with few options other than dorm food, you still have the right to be healthy. Remember that no matter how old (or young) you are, you *always* have the right to be healthy.

No Cramming for Food While You Cram for Exams

When you cram for exams, you should not be cramming in food as well. There is something about cramming in knowledge that makes you want to cram in snacks. You're thinking, you're writing, you're putting out so much energy that you want to stuff something in your mouth. I can't tell you how many times, while writing my books, I want to start munching on something, especially if I'm stuck on a thought. After six books, I realize this is part of the creative process, but I know I will be in trouble if I eat the way I did when I was in college. I remember during finals week, especially if I had to write a paper, I would knock back bagsful of sunflower seeds. It seemed to be my cramming staple, and at the end of the week, I not only found myself totally wiped out from lack of sleep but also thirsty and bloated from all the salt and oil.

The best thing you can do is have bags full of cut-up vegetables on hand, either from a salad bar or health food store. Have plenty of water available, because when you can't think, it's usually because you're dehydrated. I know even a sip of water will help me think more clearly. (It's as if I'm watering my brain!) You should drink herbal tea instead of coffee, but if you do drink coffee, try to get the water-pressed kind because it's healthier. As I mentioned before, make air-popped popcorn and spray it with Bragg's. And try my favorite snack food of all, edamame, which is boiled, salted soybeans. I wish I had known about soybeans when I was in college. Boil them on a hot plate or you can even pop a bag of them in the microwave for five minutes. Every college dorm has a microwave. They even had them when I was in college (although then it would have taken ten minutes)!

And whatever you do, stay away from those vending machines! They are the worst. Not only are they full of sugar and chemicals and caffeine, but they are expensive. Everyone on our survey who routinely ate from the vending machines put on the freshman fifteen. Every single one of them! If you're smart enough to go to college, you're smart enough to avoid the freshman fifteen.

I am a nineteen-year-old college student and I have been reading your books ever since the Total Health Makeover *came out! I have learned that in college you must learn to eat healthy and exercise. One way I do this is to shop at a grocery store to buy my own fruits and healthy snacks and soy milk. It may cost extra, but it is so much more satisfying than dorm fruit and cow's milk dispensers. Also, exercise is such a glorious stress reducer. I actually have an apartment where I can dance to my CDs, but just jogging or playing sports will help. College is a stressful time, and learning to have healthy eating and exercise habits will help you organize the rest of your life.*—KATHY FENA, CALIFORNIA

Here is a list of dorm food essentials:

Dorm Food List

Rice Dream

Soy Dream

Fruit (you can buy this or take it
from the cafeteria)

Oatmeal (instant)

Soup cups (Fantastic Foods)

Healthy corn chips, bean chips,
other salty snacks

Tuna singles (foil package
requires no can opener)

Bag of carrots

Uncle Eddie's Vegan cookies

Fruit

Cereal

Herbal teas (peppermint picks
you up; chamomile relaxes
you)

Honey

14

········

Childhood Conditions That Can Be Improved with Better Health Habits

ADD/ADHD

ADD and ADHD are disorders that started long before the '70s and '80s. Kids who suffer from them are known to benefit from the use of drugs like Ritalin. Despite this, I do not believe that we should immediately turn to prescription drugs without first investigating a child's diet, physical activity, and allergies. Medication may be the answer for some; it is certainly not the only answer. Exercise alone has been shown to be more effective than drugs like Prozac, and a strong link between allergies and ADD/ADHD has also been found. Some patients' symptoms have been alleviated by eliminating dairy, wheat, corn, yeast, soy, citrus, eggs, chocolate, peanuts, preservatives, and artificial colors from their diets Why, then, do some teachers and doctors turn a deaf ear to the benefits of exercise or diet when trying to calm a chronically hyperactive child? Fortunately this is quickly changing. A growing number of physicians believe that parents should take steps to investigate all options to improve a child's health first, and that drugs should be utilized only as a last resort. A good start toward treating ADD and ADHD is understanding what it is, its history, and its symptoms.

ADD is a behavioral syndrome that was first described by doctors in England at the beginning of the twentieth century. At the time doctors suspected that the syndrome had a hereditary link. Blaming anything other than external circumstances was radical for that time. (It is interesting to note, however, that the Industrial Revolution and the popularity of refined grains happened simultaneously.) In 1937, it was discovered that medical stimulants, such as amphetamines, often reduced the disruptive behavior of hyperactive children. In 1957, the syndrome was classified as hyperactivity, and that became the commonly accepted description of the disorder among the psychological community until the 1980s when the classification ADD/ADHD came into use. By the 1970s, more than 2,000 studies on hyperactivity had been published, although it was still commonly believed that the symptoms would disappear with the onset of puberty. Many of the researchers in this area continued to point to biological and hereditary causes for the syndrome, but others were beginning to suspect environmental causes. One of these researchers was Dr. Ben F. Feingold, who, in 1973, presented his findings to the American Medical Association, which included observations linking diet and additives with behavior and the ability to learn.

In 1972, in an address to the Canadian Psychological Association, Virginia Douglas explained a theory that shifted the focus of this syndrome from hyperactivity to deficits in sustained attention and control of impulses. Follow-up studies to her work conducted by Gabriel Weiss showed that problems with hyperactivity often lessened as children reached adolescence, but impulse and attention problems did not diminish; this was the first time the continuation of these problems into adulthood was acknowledged. In 1980, these new developments were recognized by the American Psychiatric Association and further divided into two classifications: **ADHD** (Attention Deficit with Hyperactivity and **ADD/WO** (Attention Deficit Without Hyperactivity). During the 1980s, ADHD was the single most studied childhood psychiatric disorder and probably the disorder with which children are most frequently labeled.

Currently it is estimated that 3 to 5 percent of school-age children have ADD or ADHD (as well as 2 to 4 percent of adults). While the disorders are characterized by age-inappropriate difficulties in paying attention, impulsiveness, and sometimes hyperactivity, there is no single test that can be used to diagnose them. Current medicine, however, with the use of a PET brain scan, can show metabolic differences in the ADD brain and the non-ADD brain. An ADD brain is usually less metabolically active and relies on external factors in order to gain stimulation to focus and concentrate. But extensive comprehensive evaluation is necessary to obtain an accurate diagnosis, as well as to rule out other disorders that can cause similar problems—such as anxiety disorders, mood disorders, learning disabilities, or Tourette's syndrome. Making matters even more difficult is the fact that some of these other disorders can coexist with ADD or ADHD. The first places to turn for help in obtaining a diagnosis are your physician and your child's school. Below are the American Psychiatric Association's Diagnostic Guidelines for ADD and ADHD:

A. Either (1) or (2)

   (1) *Inattention*: At least six of the following symptoms of inattention have persisted for at least six months to a degree that is maladaptive and inconsistent with developmental level:

      (a) often fails to give close attention to details or makes careless mistakes in schoolwork, work, or other activities

      (b) often has difficulty sustaining attention in tasks or play activities

      (c) often does not seem to listen to what is being said to him or her

      (d) often does not follow through on instructions and fails to finish schoolwork, chores, or duties in the workplace (not due to oppositional behavior or failure to understand instructions)

      (e) often has difficulties organizing tasks and activities

      (f) often avoids, expresses reluctance about, or has difficulties engaging in tasks that require sustained mental effort (such as schoolwork or homework)

      (g) often loses things necessary for tasks or activities (e.g., school assignments, pencils, books, tools, or toys)

      (h) is often easily distracted by extraneous stimuli

      (i) often forgetful in daily activities

   (2) *Hyperactivity-Impulsivity*: At least five of the following symptoms of hyperactivity-impulsivity have persisted for at least six months to a degree that is maladaptive and inconsistent with developmental level:

   Hyperactivity

      (a) often fidgets with hands or feet or squirms in seat

      (b) leaves seat in classroom or in other situations in which remaining seated is expected

(c) often runs about or climbs excessively in situations where it is inappropriate (in adolescents or adults, may be limited to subjective feelings of restlessness)

(d) often has difficulty playing or engaging in leisure activities quietly

(e) is always "on the go" or acts as if "driven by a motor"

(f) often talks excessively

Impulsiveness

(g) often blurts out answers to questions before the questions have been completed

(h) often has difficulty waiting in lines or awaiting turn in games or group situations

(i) often interrupts or intrudes on others (e.g., butts into others' conversations or games)

B. Some symptoms that caused impairment were present before age seven.

C. Some symptoms that cause impairment are present in two or more settings (e.g., at school, work, and at home).

D. There must be clear evidence of clinically significant impairment in social, academic, or occupational functioning.

E. Does not occur exclusively during the course of a Pervasive Developmental Disorder, Schizophrenia or other Psychotic Disorder, and is not better accounted for by Mood Disorder, Anxiety Disorder, Dissociative Disorder, or a Personality Disorder.

Genetic defects or metabolic disorders can both be causes of learning disabilities. While there is no cure for the genetic causes, you need to understand the basic cell and brain function to see why it is possible for metabolic disorders to cause learning disabilities. Each cell in our body has its own metabolism and performs various functions that are beneficial to the body as a whole. The process of cell metabolism is dependent upon more than 2,000 enzymes which the cells produce. When toxins that have entered the body through the air, water, or food destroy these enzymes, the cells will begin to malfunction and be unable to perform some of the processes that they are needed for.

Psychostimulants such as Ritalin, Adderall, and Dexedrine are the medications most commonly used to control the problems brought on by ADD or ADHD. While there are many documented cases of these medications helping children suffering from these syndromes, it must be noted that medications such as Ritalin are classified as Class II controlled substances, which means they are noted for "high abuse potential." Currently there is a great deal of controversy about whether ADD and ADHD are overdiagnosed syndromes as well as about the overprescription of drugs such as Ritalin. As I stated earlier, the problems of children suffering with ADD or ADHD are very real and very serious. But there is considerable and growing support for addressing these problems through changes in diet and exercise. It seems obvious to me that these options should be examined before moving on to decisions involving medication. There are also numerous testimonials from parents who have seen their children's extensive behavioral problems dissipate after they discovered food allergies or reactions to additives as the cause and removed these foods and additives from the children's diets.

After seeing the results of THM on me, I decided to incorporate it seriously with my family. The first thing I did was take my son off all refined sugar. I decided to start with this step because he has always been a "difficult child." I had been told by other mothers, some of whom have ADHD children, that my son was also ADHD. I had a mother get the forms used to test these children for ADHD. By those forms, my son did have it. I still never believed that something was "wrong" with my son.

After about three weeks of being off refined sugar and getting it out of his system, Zachary was all of the sudden "Here." I don't know how else to explain it other than that. He's always lived in his own little world, but now, I have him here with us. His behavior at school is so much better as well. I haven't gotten a phone call home from the principals office in months. He's also starting to bloom socially where as before he didn't connect with the other kids.

I just recently received a letter from his school asking if I would consent to my son being tested for "giftedness." They sent home a checklist of twenty-eight possible reasons why they feel my son is gifted. Out of twenty-eight of those, there were twenty-six checked!!! I honestly don't believe this would have been recognized if I had not taken refined sugar out of his diet.

Once in a while, he is given candy at school (against my instructions). It is very obvious to me when this happens because his behavior shows it. It's actually amazing to see it happen. I can count on the next three days being tough on everyone. After three days of no sugar and lots of whole foods, he's back to normal.

Thanks Marilu. I can't even begin to express to you how grateful I am for what you've done. I hope our story will be able to help other families out there in the same situation. Maybe they'll read it and decided to try changing the diet before considering other measures.—ALLISON MERRIMAN, TENNESSEE

Allergies/Asthma

We tend to associate allergic reactions with hay fever, hives, runny eyes, a rash, or, in the extreme, asthma. But the truth is that they can take many forms, including headaches, stomachaches, joint or muscle aches, sleep problems, and even behavioral and learning problems. This is not to say that every time our children have a stomachache or headache they're experiencing an allergy or food sensitivity. But when such symptoms continue over time, you should certainly examine them and consider the possibility that your child is suffering an allergic reaction to factors either in his diet or in his environment. One of the main reasons children suffer from allergies is that their immune system may not be functioning at maximum capability. The use of various nutrients, taken in correct amounts, can help to strengthen the immune system against natural irritants such as pollen, dust, and mold.

It is estimated that as many as 6 percent of American children suffer from food allergies. These children carry allergic antibodies (Immunoglobulin E) that cause them to overreact to ordinary harmless food. Food allergens, which are the parts of foods that cause the problem, are usually proteins, and they are responsible for up to 90 percent of allergic reactions. The most common of these are the proteins in eggs, cow's milk, peanuts, wheat, soy, fish, shellfish, and tree nuts. As the body tries to fight off the allergens, symptoms begin to appear. The most common sites for these symptoms are the mouth (swelling of the tongue, swelling or itching of the lips), the digestive tract (vomiting, cramps, diarrhea), the skin (rash, hives, or eczema), or the air passages (wheezing, breathing problems). A severe allergic reaction is known as *anaphylaxis*, the first signs of which can be a feeling of warmth, flushing, tingling in the mouth, or a red rash. In the most severe cases, a drop in blood pressure or loss of consciousness can occur. Anaphylaxis requires immediate medical attention and can be reversed by an injection of epinephrine or antihistamines. As children grow older they may outgrow certain food allergies, except for peanut or tree-nut allergies.

Food intolerance is sometimes mistaken for a food allergy. Food intolerance is an abnormal physical response to a food or food additive, but is not an allergic reaction and does not involve the immune system. The most common of these is lactose intolerance, in which a child lacks the proper enzymes to break down the sugars in milk. Sometimes food intolerance may be a reaction to the chemicals or additives in foods. The additives that most frequently cause intolerance reactions are aspartame, Yellow Dye No. 5, Red Dye No. 3, MSG, nitrates, and sulfites. Sulfites can be a particular problem for children with asthma. Sulfites can give off a gas (sulfur dioxide) that can irritate the lungs and cause severe constriction. Because of this, the FDA has now banned spray-on preservatives in fresh fruits and vegetables, but they are still used in other foods.

Asthma affects 8 to 12 percent of children in the United States and has increased here and in other developed countries over the past fifteen years at the same time that other lung diseases, such as tuberculosis and pneumonia, have significantly decreased.

Asthma is a chronic inflammatory disease of the lungs that can be triggered by allergies, exercise, viral infections, or smoke. Its cause is not known, though it often seems to be an inherited condition. During an asthma attack, the muscles that line the airways constrict and tighten. The airways become inflamed and are further narrowed by the mucus that builds up; this causes the muscles that line the airways to tighten. This can cause coughing, wheezing, increased heart rate, and shortness of breath. Such symptoms can make asthma attacks very frightening and sometimes life-threatening. Among chronic illnesses, it is the most frequently named for kids who are admitted to hospital emergency rooms. In fact, during a recent visit to a children's hospital emergency room, I was amazed to find out that 6 out of 9 patients were there for asthma. It is the number one reason for children who repeatedly miss school.

Diagnosing asthma can be complicated by the fact that symptoms can differ greatly in children. With some, there may be coughing at night that is not manifested during the day. Some kids get frequent chest colds that don't seem to go away. Your physician will use various methods, including allergy tests, blood tests, and chest X-rays, to diagnose asthma and will undoubtedly want to obtain an extensive family medical history as well.

If your child suffers from asthma, you should be aware that some foods might provoke an attack. Studies show that diets which are high in dairy and meat cause more asthma attacks than vegetarian diets, simply because there are more allergy-causing components in dairy and meat. Vegetable oils such as corn, safflower and sunflower, which are all high in omega-6 fatty acids, should also be avoided because they can promote inflammation.

Diabetes

Diabetes exists in two basic forms. Type 1, usually referred to as juvenile diabetes, is caused by a defect in the immune system that destroys the beta cells in the pancreas that produce insulin. Artificial insulin must be given to those suffering from this in order to normalize their blood sugar levels. Children with Type 1 diabetes are usually not obese; they may, in fact, show signs of weight loss. The typical symptoms of diabetes—thirst and frequent urination—may exist only for a short time and then recur periodically. Ketones will show up in urine when it is tested. The high blood sugar levels that result from diabetes can ultimately result in damage to the nerves, organs, and blood vessels. This damage may take the form of heart disease, blindness, kidney failure, or poor circulation, which can be responsible for infections in the feet or legs.

Type 2 diabetes, which has traditionally been known as adult-onset diabetes, is a form of the disease in which the body produces enough insulin but the individual cells become resistant to it. There has been a marked increase in cases of Type 2 diabetes in children in recent years. Children with Type 2 diabetes are most likely to be overweight. Sugar may appear in their urine but not ketones. They may not show any signs of thirst or increased urination, but 40 to 80 percent of them will have at least one parent with the disease. In 90 percent of these children, dark shiny patches on the skin, usually between the fingers or toes, can be seen. Since an increase in hormone levels can cause insulin resistance, it follows that Type 2 diabetes in children often occurs during puberty. The American Diabetes Association suggests that children older than ten (or younger, if puberty has already occurred) whose body mass index is greater than the eighty-fifth percentile (or whose weight is 120 percent of the ideal for their height) be screened for Type 2 diabetes if at least two of the following factors also exist:

(1) A family history of Type 2 diabetes in a first- or second-degree relative

(2) The presence of any of the signs of insulin resistance; these may include conditions such as acanthosis nigricans (hyperpigmentation and wartlike growths in the folds of the skin), multiple cysts in the ovaries, high blood pressure, or blood fat disorders

(3) An African-American, Hispanic, American Indian, Asian, or Pacific Islander ethnic background

The ideal diet for people with diabetes is low in fat, salt, and added sugars. Ideally, it will be high in complex carbohydrates, such as whole grains and whole grain breads, cereals, and pasta, as well as fruits and vegetables. Portion size can also be essential in order to keep weight down.

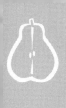

15

· · · · · · · · · · ·

Thinking Outside
the (Toy) Box

L et's have some fun!

We've done it all. We've discussed what goes into our children's bodies and what goes into their minds in terms of our input and influence. Now let's talk about what stimulates their minds and gets them to think in more creative ways. Let's get them to color out of the lines, explore what's not on the map, think outside the box.

As you probably know by now, I grew up in a very noisy, creative family. Because there were six kids, my parents had to do many things to keep us entertained and in line, but they also looked for opportunities to stimulate our imaginations and to teach us how to think. And one of my favorites among the things they used to do was to make up games you could not find anywhere else.

My father loved to challenge our minds with special games he made up that always seemed better than any that came in a box. I so appreciate the way my parents raised the six of us, and so I have always looked for ways to pass on to my children the sense of fun and adventure and love of learning that my parents gave to my brothers and sisters and me. I am always looking for any opportunity to stimulate my children's minds and to get them to think in more creative ways.

Who When They Were Little

One day while I was giving my kids a bath and they wanted to play a game, I thought, "Here is a perfect opportunity to give them a bath, play a game, and at the same time teach them something about their family history." They, of course, knew all of their aunts and uncles and were naturally curious about what they were all like when they were little kids. I had a very colorful family and it was a wonderful way to grow up. The six of us had very different personalities and different tastes, especially when we were small. So my boys and I made up a game during bath time called Who When They Were Little. Nicky and Joey would pick a category (for example, "Birthday Cakes") and I would say, "Okay, who when they were little liked coconut cake? Who when they were little liked chocolate cake?" and they would have to guess which of my siblings was the correct answer. With every category, my boys would learn a lot about what their aunts and uncles were like when they were children. You can play this game with your children and use members of your family or friends or anyone that you knew when they were young. You can pick different categories, from favorite animals to favorite TV shows to birthday parties to crazy school stories to, even, injuries. My boys know more about my brothers and sisters than some of their own children know or even more than my brothers and sisters remember about their own lives. I have always been the family historian, and having a good memory, I recall a lot about my childhood (more than I have ever really needed to!). Anyway, Who When They Were Little is a great game to play with your children that teaches them about your family at the same time.

The Stair Game

This game is played on a staircase; the players sit on the top step and each step represents a different subject. Let's say the first step is the spelling step and I give each player an age-appropriate word that he must spell. The next step might be math and the next one science, but whatever the subject, it is always possible to ask a question that is suitable for the age of the child. My boys are two years apart in school, and because they are learning different things, I always make the question relevant to their experience. In fact, I have played this game with children as young as three years old; you can always find something in each subject that a child can relate to. You can make one of the steps about colors or holidays or *Sesame Street*—whatever it takes to challenge the players and make them think. The rules of the game are that if a child gets an answer right, he moves to the next step, and if he gets it wrong, he remains on his current step. When a player gets down to the last three steps, he enters the bonus round, and he can pick his favorite subject from the categories you have already used (or he can pick a category not used). This last move helps level the playing field because some kids like science better or math or colors or physics or geography or history. It's like a kid's *Jeopardy* in a way because you can make a step represent any subject, even family history or popular television shows. My boys love to play this game whenever their friends are over, and because the game feels fair, kids of all ages can play together. The only challenge is that *you* have to know the answers because *you* have to make up the questions.

I Went to the Store

This is a game my uncle made up when we were kids. My uncle was a real character. He lived upstairs from us with ten cats, two dogs, two birds, a skunk, 150 fish, and his friend Charles. He taught art at our grammar school and after school ran art classes in his home. He was also the neighborhood astrologer and ran a cat hospital on our roof. He was my mother's youngest brother and they obviously came from a very entrepreneurial family because my mother, like her younger brother, was multitalented. She ran a dancing school in our garage and a beauty shop in our kitchen. (And people wonder how I ended up in show business!)

Anyway, this game is played with any age group, but it's better if the kids can print or write their answers. It can be played with any number of people, but at least three are required. Each person needs a sheet of paper, a pencil, and an idea of a store they went to, what they bought, what they did with their purchase, and what was the outcome.

Let's say I'm playing the game and my piece of paper is in front of me. So I write, "I went to the pet store." I fold the paper so that no one can see what I wrote and pass it to the person on my right. At the same time the person on my left gives me her piece of paper, and of course I can't read what she wrote either. Now I write, "I bought a dog." I fold the paper and pass it to my right. Again, I get another piece of paper from the person on my left. I write, "I took him home," fold the paper, pass it, and receive from the left. I write, "He poo-pooed on the carpet." Now everyone is finished, and as I unfold the paper in front of me, it reads, "I went to the jewelry store. I bought a TV. I gave it to my brother Lorin. He poo-pooed on the carpet."

You will be amazed at how the jumbled answers really do fit together to make funny stories that almost make sense. Although the game is called I Went to the Store, you can also name a place you went to (i.e., Disneyland) in order to make a different kind of scenario. My kids love this game because you never know what to expect (kind of like my uncle's house!).

The Memory Game

I have always wanted my children to have great memories, because I have one, and I have always been grateful for it. In fact, it is something I have become famous for. I often go on talk shows and have people give me a specific date; then I will tell them what day of the week it was and what I was doing on that day. I developed a good memory because, as a child, I loved to relive events in my mind. I actually invented a technique for this in the first grade. I would lie in bed at night saying, "Okay, what did I do a week ago today? What did I do two weeks ago today? Three weeks ago?" And so on. I would actually relive my days, and this became my device for falling asleep at night as well as a way of developing my memory. Memory is like any other muscle in your body. It needs to be exercised. And if you do exercise it, it is amazing how much stronger and more responsive it will become.

My father always used to say that every event has three parts to it—anticipation, participation, and recollection and the greatest of these is recollection. My parents used to throw these incredible family parties when I was a child, and we all anticipated them and talked about them for weeks before. In the middle of the party, we were able to participate in the moment and appreciate that the event was actually taking place. But as my father said, the recollection, the talking about the party the next morning or reliving it with one another the following week, that was the best part of all. To this day, I can go back in time and think about a specific party and remember it in detail.

Anyway, because I wanted my children to have good memories, I figured I would start when they were very little. I helped them become aware of the three parts to every event—the anticipation, the participation, and the recollection. For example, when we were going to my sister's house, I would say, "Oh we're going to go to Aunt JoAnn's house. And what are we going to see there?" And I'd remind them of what we were going to see. Then, while we were there, we saw the things we had talked about, and afterward we relived the experience. My kids got very good at remembering events. People are surprised that to this day my boys remember details from when they were really young. They love to remember things, so they made up a game called the Memory Game in which they have me test them on the details of a person, place, event, or experience. For example, we recently finished a twenty-two-city road tour and I'll ask them, "In what city did this happen? In what city did that happen?" It is a constant way of stimulating their memories and making them relate certain things to other things. That's what memory is. It is relating one thing to many things or many things to one thing. I am always asking my boys to take in their surroundings and then describe things with their eyes closed. I want them to be conscious and aware of what it is they are in the middle of experiencing, and by doing that, I am training them to have good memories. The Memory Game can be about anything you do, from your family vacations to different holidays to birthday parties, different grades, different teachers, any experience that your children have, even as simple as their day at school. The best thing about the Memory Game is that it can be played anywhere, at any time, as long as you remember to have fun!

Creating Your Own Bedtime Stories

The Story Game

The Story Game is a game I invented to get my kids more actively involved than they can be when simply listening to a story. I ask them to give me six elements that will have to show up in the story. (It reminds me of being in the fourth grade and having to find a way to use the weekly ten spelling words in one paragraph.) For example, I'll say, "Joey, give me a color. Nicky, give me a superhero. Joey, give me a city." We go on and on until we have six different elements. (It can be anything—a food, a toy, a song, and so on.) We then proceed to make up a story, working those elements into the plot. One of us starts the story, and at some point that person "passes" the storytelling responsibility to another person. This continues until all the words have been included and the story has come to a natural conclusion. We usually play the Story Game at bedtime because we can play with the lights out. It is a joy to witness how inventive your children can be, and I feel it is a wonderful way to stimulate their imaginations as they ready themselves to enter the sleep state. I like to believe that I am not only helping to develop their storytelling abilities, but who knows, one of them may turn out to be the next Tom Clancy, John Irving, or (yikes!) Stephen King.

First Line, Last Line

This idea came from my old improv days when members of the audience would shout out two lines to be used as the first and last in a sketch. The way my kids and I play it, one person comes up with a sentence that begins a story and another person comes up with a sentence that ends the story, and usually I have to come up with the story in between. My boys love to pick two lines that have nothing to do with each other and watch me suffer as I try to connect the two diverse ideas. This is a great bedtime-story technique when you don't have a lot of time but still want to get the job done. Be careful, though—this can backfire when the two lines are so far apart that making up a story that makes sense takes twenty minutes or longer.

Mad Libs

This is another version of the game you play with pencil and paper, but we play it out loud. You start a story and stop on a word that your child then has to fill in. It is fun to let your story twist and turn with each answer, and you never know where the story will end up because the choices your kids make are never what you expect. For example, I could say, "Once upon a time, there was a little (blank)"; I am expecting one of my kids to shout out "boy," and instead he says "octopus"! It is best if you take the journey with your kids and let their choices determine the story. I played this game with my son's pre-K class, and it was amazing to hear how the kids filled in the blanks. You can play it with any age, of course, and as they get older you can call for the word in a more sophisticated way—i.e., noun, adverb, adjective, etc.

ABC Song

Sometimes my boys want a song before they go to sleep, and instead of practicing my show tunes (which by this time they are sick of), they insist on my version of the ABC Song. I start to sing the song, but because almost every letter could also be a word, I allow any letter to launch me into a different song, thereby making it impossible to get through all of the ABCs. For example, I sing "ABCDEFGHI love you, you love me . . ." and then I start again. "ABCDEFGHIJKL is for the way you look at me . . ." Again I try "ABC,c,c,c,c,a,a,a, a minor . . ." and so on. You never know on what letter the new song will take off because almost every letter lends itself to some kind of detour. The idea is for us to get through the alphabet once. But believe me, it can get crazier and crazier trying to get through the ABC song because, like every sitcom second banana, each letter wants its own spin-off! It usually ends with my getting through the song completely exhausted, with a final "Next time won't you sing with me . . . 'a name I call myself' . . ."

16

· · · · · · · · · · · ·

Just for Kids:
Puzzles, Games, and More

O ne of the best ways to teach your children anything is to make a game out of it. (In fact, to this day I can tell you the valances of the elements because of a rhyme I made up. And my brother, Lorin, can recite all fifty states in alphabetical order in less than twenty seconds.)

The following is a series of word searches, crossword puzzles, anagrams, and other interactive games to help your child learn about nutrition. Just think while you're cooking, they can be coloring!

HIDDEN WHOLE FOODS TO EAT

Find the foods that are "good for you" and circle them.
They're hidden up, down, across, diagonally, and in reverse. Have fun!

```
R Y E L A E M T A O S T R A W B E R R I E S
O B E A N S I O L L Q T O F U E C I O R E N
D R T L A S R A I I U Z R T W N I C Z I W I
A O N I O N S Y M V A N A A F U P E R N S S
C C Q A Z O A B E E S A N I L R S R R O O I
O C U C U M B E R S H U G R A P E S O M Y A
V O B N S E M G K G T S E B N B L E Z L B R
A L B O R L E G A B B A C H I C K E N A E E
F I S H R M Y S L Y K A I Z Y M L D L S A W
W V S N I A R G A E I R R E Z U L S T U N O
S E A W E E D A S L W K N A N L B R A N S L
X O R S G H H Y L R I O W R R P M A N G O F
M I S O A T S A I A H T O M A T O E S W P I
A L K Y J T I P T B Z C R A A E C U T T E L
T U R K E Y D A N A N A B R E A D S Q W A U
N B R E A D A P E A C H E S H C A N I P S A
O T B W B Y R E L E C A E P U O L A T N A C
T U O R P S L E S S U R B S U G A R A P S A
```

Asparagus	Corn	Lime	Rice
Avocado	Cucumbers	Mango	Rye
Bananas	Eggs	Miso	Salmon
Beets	Figs	Oatmeal	Seaweed
Berries	Fish	Okra	Soy
Breads	Garlic	Olives	Soybeans
Brown rice	Grain	Onions	Spice
Brussel sprout	Grapes	Oranges	Spinach
Cabbage	Honey	Papaya	Squash
Cantaloupe	Kale	Peaches	Strawberries
Carrots	Kiwi	Peas	Tomatoes
Cauliflower	Lemons	Plum	Tuna
Celery	Lentils	Prune	Turkey
Chicken	Lettuce	Radish	Yams

VEGETABLE VITAMIN SOUP

UNSCRAMBLE THESE DELICIOUS LETTERS TO
FIND OUT WHAT'S IN THE SOUP. COLOR EACH
COMPLETE WORD THE COLOR OF THE VEGETABLE.
ENJOY . . .

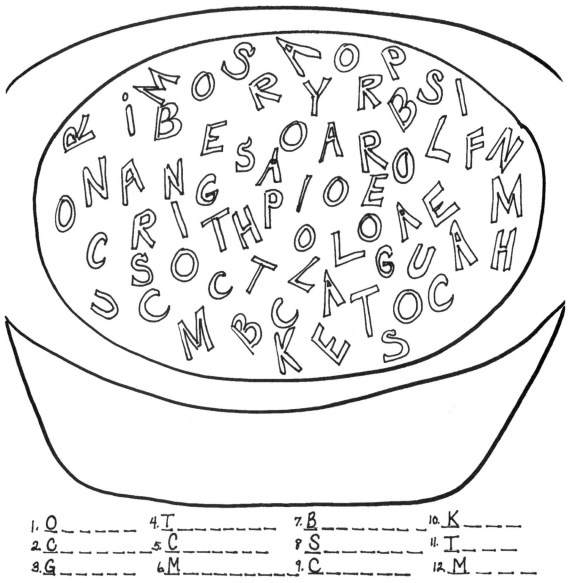

1. O _ _ _ _ _
2. C _ _ _ _ _
3. G _ _ _ _ _
4. T _ _ _ _ _ _
5. C _ _ _ _ _
6. M _ _ _ _ _ _
7. B _ _ _ _ _ _ _
8. S _ _ _ _ _
9. C _ _ _ _ _
10. K _ _ _ _
11. T _ _ _ _
12. M _ _ _

WORD SEARCH

Find all of these healthy foods in the puzzle below.

C	A	L	C	I	U	M	R	I	A	F
A	C	K	M	R	N	T	I	P	I	P
R	D	U	F	O	T	I	C	B	E	R
B	A	N	A	N	A	U	E	A	K	O
O	Z	U	B	A	L	R	O	R	O	T
H	W	T	R	Y	Q	F	T	L	H	E
Y	O	S	O	A	O	I	A	E	C	I
D	D	P	C	P	M	S	T	Y	I	N
R	A	I	C	A	Z	H	O	A	T	S
A	C	N	O	P	S	A	P	S	R	L
T	O	A	L	Q	T	E	E	I	A	S
E	V	C	I	M	E	M	E	N	T	N
S	A	H	E	C	U	Z	U	D	S	I
P	Z	A	I	G	W	T	A	F	S	A
Q	L	R	E	B	M	U	C	U	C	R
S	E	L	B	A	T	E	G	E	V	G

1. Carbohydrates	8. Broccoli	15. Cucumber	22. Pasta
2. Protein	9. Fish	16. Legumes	23. Nuts
3. Fat	10. Potato	17. Papaya	24. Vegetables
4. Calcium	11. Barley	18. Spinach	25. Tofu
5. Iron	12. Oats	19. Oatmeal	26. Soy
6. Fiber	13. Seeds	20. Rice	27. Banana
7. Fruit	14. Avocado	21. Artichoke	

THE UNHEALTHY WORD SEARCH

Can you find all of the unhealthy words below?

C	H	O	L	E	S	T	E	R	O	L
R	A	G	U	S	P	K	O	Q	O	R
S	D	F	A	S	T	F	O	O	D	O
M	D	T	F	R	U	I	T	T	R	L
O	I	A	V	E	G	G	I	E	S	O
K	T	E	O	A	I	R	Y	M	G	C
I	I	M	A	F	Q	N	R	I	S	L
N	V	S	F	I	G	R	E	L	L	A
G	E	S	S	L	M	N	R	A	I	
R	S	N	E	H	C	S	E	D	M	C
E	W	A	F	J	W	D	O	P	O	I
T	A	E	H	O	H	E	Y	D	L	F
T	T	B	C	A	N	D	Y	O	A	I
O	E	Y	L	O	H	O	C	L	A	T
B	R	O	W	N	S	U	G	A	R	R
M	K	S	A	X	A	S	T	R	M	A

Unhealthy

Additives	Brown Sugar	Cholesterol	Smoking
Alcohol	Caffeine	Fast Food	Sugar
Artificial Color	Candy	Meat	Soda

Now find the five healthy words that are not listed:

1. _ _ _ _

2. _ _ _ _ _ _

3. _ _ _ _ _ _

4. _ _ _ _ _ _ _ _

5. _ _ _ _ _ _ _

THE GOOD FOOD PYRAMID

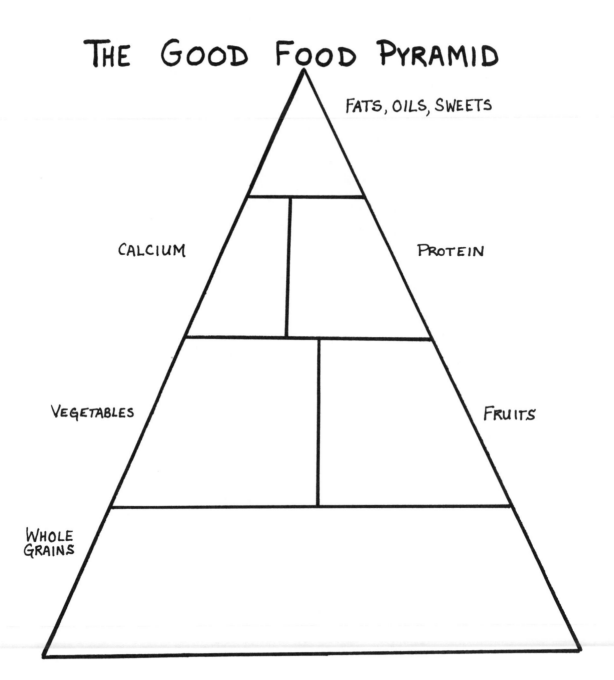

FATS, OILS, SWEETS

CALCIUM

PROTEIN

VEGETABLES

FRUITS

WHOLE
GRAINS

PYRAMID PUZZLER

SEE IF YOU CAN FIND THE CORRECT BLOCK OF THE PYRAMID TO PLACE THESE WONDERFUL THINGS TO EAT AND WRITE THEM IN. HAVE FUN!

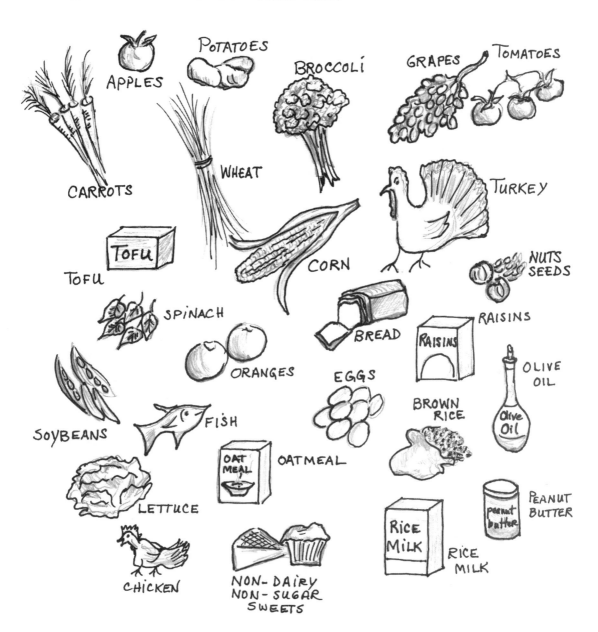

APPLES

POTATOES

BROCCOLI

GRAPES

TOMATOES

CARROTS

WHEAT

TURKEY

TOFU

CORN

NUTS SEEDS

SPINACH

BREAD

RAISINS

ORANGES

EGGS

OLIVE OIL

SOYBEANS

FISH

BROWN RICE

OATMEAL

LETTUCE

PEANUT BUTTER

RICE MILK

CHICKEN

NON-DAIRY NON-SUGAR SWEETS

COLORFUL FRUITS

FRUITS COME IN MANY BEAUTIFUL DELICIOUS COLORS.
CHECK THE BOX WITH THE COLORS THAT MATCH THESE FRUITS.
SOME FRUITS COME IN MORE THAN ONE COLOR.

	RED	YELLOW	GREEN	ORANGE	PURPLE	PINK
1. apples						
2. oranges						
3. grapes						
4. pineapple						
5. bananas						
6. pears						
7. cantaloupe						
8. peaches						
9. plums						
10. watermelon						

How Does Your Garden Grow?

LESSONS ON GROWING YOUR VERY OWN VEGETABLES!

LET'S MAKE
GREEN ONIONS

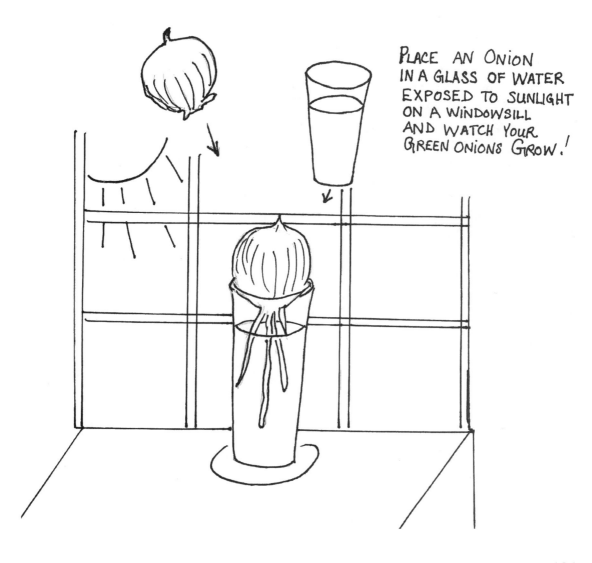

PLACE AN ONION IN A GLASS OF WATER EXPOSED TO SUNLIGHT ON A WINDOWSILL AND WATCH YOUR GREEN ONIONS GROW.!

WHAT'S IN YOUR REFRIGERATOR?

SEE IF YOU CAN MATCH A HEALTHIER FOOD IN
THE GOOD FRIDGE WITH A FOOD IN THE BAD FRIDGE
AND DRAW A LINE CONNECTING THE TWO SIMILAR FOODS.

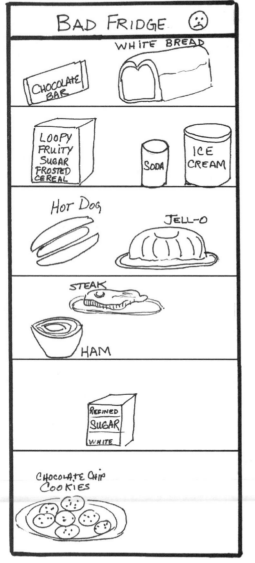

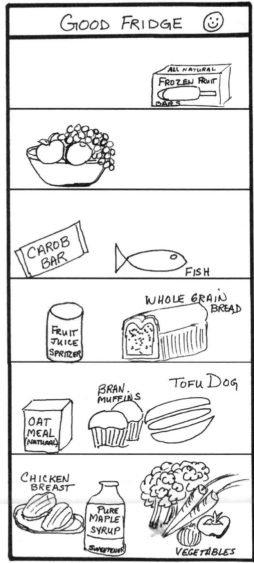

VITAMIN A

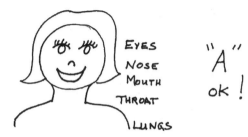

EYES
NOSE
MOUTH
THROAT
LUNGS

"A" ok!

VITAMIN A HELPS PROTECT THE MUCOUS MEMBRANES IN THE NOSE, MOUTH, THROAT, AND LUNGS. IT HELPS FIGHT INFECTION AND IS GOOD FOR HEALTHY SKIN AND EYESIGHT.

MATCH THE CORRECT PICTURE AND WORD TO GET TO KNOW THESE NUTRITIOUS FOODS TO BE "A" OK!

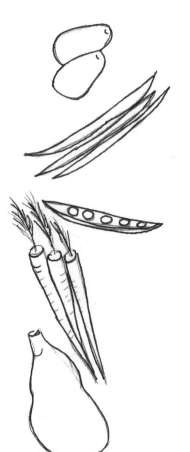

CARROTS

SQUASH

AVOCADOS

SPINACH

TOMATOES

BEET GREENS

APRICOTS

GREEN BEANS

PEAS

PEACHES

ALFALFA SPROUTS

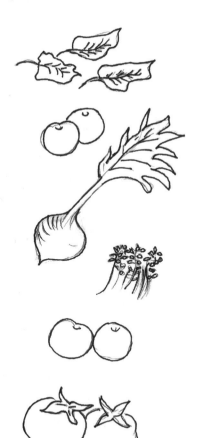

HOW DO YOU LIKE YOUR FOOD?

Give It a Rating
(Least Favorite 1 to Favorite 10)

BREAKFAST	LUNCH

DINNER	SNACK

Keep this daily food diary to see how well you've been eating. Remember, 5 fruits and vegetables a day!

UNSCRAMBLE

Good for You—Bad for You

Good for You		Bad for You	
CLORIBCO	_____	ARDYI	_____
RAROCTS	_____	ATEM	_____
YHLTEHA	_____	GRUSA	_____
HNAIPSC	_____	TATEUARSD ATF	_____
GEANROS	_____	DITEVSIDA	_____
SPLPAE	_____	HEMCAILSC	_____
REPGAS	_____	SPEEVRVTIRASE	_____
XRIECEES	_____	FFEECNAI	_____
PELES	_____	YANDC	_____
TENORPI	_____	STAF FODO	_____

Good for You

BROCCOLI
CARROTS
HEALTHY
SPINACH
ORANGES
APPLES
GRAPES
EXERCISE
SLEEP
PROTEIN

Bad for You

DAIRY
MEAT
SUGAR
SATURATED FAT
ADDITIVES
CHEMICALS
PRESERVATIVES
CAFFEINE
CANDY
FAST FOOD

FAVORITE FRUITS AND VEGETABLES

Do this nutritious crossword puzzle to find out just how good these fruits and vegetables are for you. Have fun! When you have finished, have one of your favorites to eat. Yum!

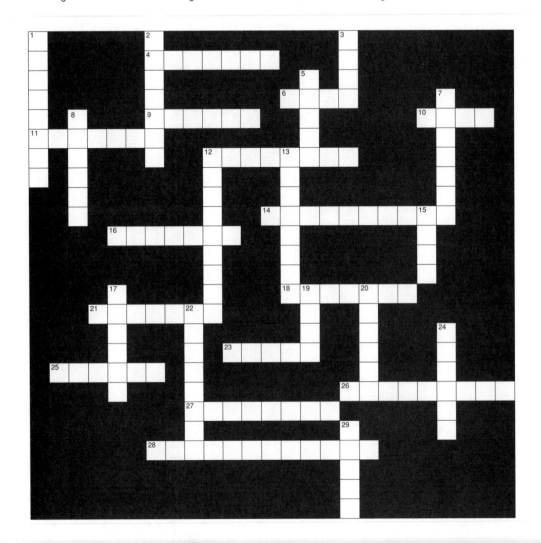

Across

4. This delicious fruit, grown in California, is high in vitamin A, which helps your body's tissues grow and repair. Let's have guacamole.

6. A sweet orange potato that is high in potassium, which is good for your muscles and helps you grow.

9. A breakfast citrus fruit high in vitamin C and bioflavonoids. It is good protection against colds.

10. A green leafy vegetable that's part of the cabbage family. It's high in vitamin A and helps prevent bone fractures.

11. A sweet orange and yellow fruit with soft skin.

This yummy one has riboflavin, which keeps your hair shiny and your cheeks rosy.

12. A popular vegetable you love to eat. It can be made into French fries. It's high in potassium and good for your heart and skin.

14. A breakfast melon high in vitamin C. It helps you heal and builds red blood cells.

16. A sweet yellow fruit that you peel and eat. It's high in potassium, which keeps your skin healthy and gives you lots of energy.

18. A green leafy vegetable that tastes great cooked or in your salad. It's high in iron and keeps you strong.

21. A green leafy vegetable, rich in vitamin K, which helps your blood to clot normally and your liver to work properly.

23. A light green fiber-rich fruit that helps you digest your food. It has iodine, which helps you grow and develop.

25. A red fruit that comes in bunches. It's high in vitamin C, which gives you energy and keeps you healthy.

26. A highly nutritious vegetable that's green and looks a little like a tree. It has calcium to build strong bones and teeth.

27. This green vegetable comes in a bunch with flowery tips. It's a good source of sodium, which helps keep your cells hydrated.

28. A sweet snack high in vitamin A. This red fun fruit makes your skin healthy. Berry-licious.

Down

1. This very special green legume is good for you. It's also high in protein to help your body build tissues.

2. A crunchy orange vegetable that's rich in vitamin A. It helps keep your skin healthy and is good for your eyesight.

3. This sweet green or purple fruit is often eaten dried. It contains bromelain, and helps fight cancer.

5. This red and green tropical fruit with a golden inside is a good antioxidant that has the ability to destroy free radicals that eat healthy cells.

7. A crispy, round leafy vegetable that's purple or yellow-green. Coleslaw is made from this calcium-rich food.

8. This fruit grows in bunches and can be purple, red, or green. It's high in vitamin C, which equals energy!

12. A very sweet Hawaiian tropical fruit which is high in vitamin C. The bromelain it contains helps treat bruises.

13. A ripe, juicy red fruit that most people think is a vegetable. It's rich in vitamin C and great in salads.

15. A round, sweet purple fruit. It has bioflavonoids, which help strengthen the capillaries.

17. A crunchy green vegetable with a long stem. It tastes great with peanut butter and contains sulfur, the mineral for glossy hair and a beautiful complexion.

19. These green pods are a good source of vitamin A, which helps protect against infection. They also contain vitamin B_{12}, which is good for your skin, hair, nails, and eyesight.

20. This fruit, eaten every day, keeps the doctor away. It has magnesium, which helps your bones grow and muscles work.

22. A cool, crunchy vegetable that's long and green. It's great in salad and can be made into pickles.

24. A delicious tropical fruit that is very high in potassium and vitamin C. It's great for helping digest food.

29. A red root vegetable that tastes great cold in your salad or as a soup. It's a good source of vitamin A, which makes your skin soft.

Answer Key

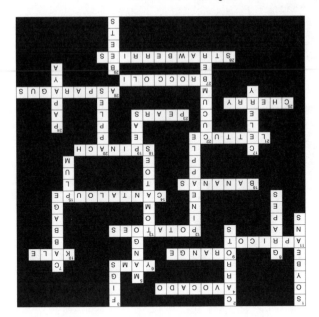

17

· · · · · · · · · · · ·

Kid-Friendly Recipes

O kay. Let's eat!

Here are over 100 recipes to prove to you that healthy food can be delicious. These recipes are not only tasty and good for you, but they are also kid-friendly and easy to make. When I polled children all over the country and asked, "What are your five favorite foods?" I took their answers to heart and gathered together the healthy versions of all their favorites and more. You will find plenty of fruits, veggies, whole grains, legumes, and lean proteins—all of the good stuff we've been talking about throughout this book. Even the recipes that bend the rules a little (flour products) are the healthiest versions possible. So go ahead. Get the kids in the kitchen and have fun!

B.E.S.T. of Health!

BREAKFAST

Energy Packin' Pancakes

Makes 4 servings

1 cup soy or rice milk
4 cage-free eggs, separated
1 cup unbleached flour
Dash of salt

1 tablespoon Sucanat or
  maple sugar
1½ teaspoons baking powder
Cooking oil for frying

Preheat a griddle or large skillet over medium-low heat. Beat the soy or rice milk and egg yolks in a small bowl. Mix the dry ingredients in a medium bowl. Beat the egg whites with a whisk or an electric mixer until fluffy. Add the soy milk and yolk mixture to the dry ingredients and stir until blended. Gently fold in the egg whites.

Put approximately 1 teaspoon oil in the skillet. When it's hot, add the batter, 1 tablespoon at a time. Cook the pancakes until lightly brown on the bottom, approximately 3 to 5 minutes. Flip and cook until golden, about 1 to 2 minutes more.

VARIATIONS

Blueberry Pancakes: Add 1 cup fresh or frozen organic blueberries to the batter as the last ingredient. If using frozen, do not defrost before adding, and cook the pancakes a little more slowly since they have a tendency to burn.

Banana Pancakes: After dropping the batter onto the pan, place a few ¼-inch-thick organic banana slices directly onto the surface of the batter and cook as directed.

Buckwheat Pancakes: Use 1¼ cups soy or rice milk; 4 cage-free eggs, separated; 1 cup buckwheat flour; dash of salt; and 2 tablespoons Sucanat or maple sugar. Follow the same cooking and mixing instructions as for Energy Packin' Pancakes.

Willy's Wacky Waffles

Makes 4 servings

Canola oil cooking spray for waffle iron

2 cups unbleached flour

½ teaspoon salt

3 teaspoons baking powder

2 tablespoons Sucanat or maple sugar

1½ cups soy or rice milk

2 cage-free eggs

4 tablespoons soy margarine,
    melted and cooled

1 teaspoon vanilla

Spray the waffle iron with oil and preheat. Combine the dry ingredients in a large bowl. Mix the soy milk and eggs in a medium bowl. Stir in the soy margarine and vanilla. Add the wet ingredients to the dry ones and stir until blended. Pour on the waffle iron and cook until golden brown on each side.

VARIATION

Banana-Split Waffles: Top a waffle with 1 tablespoon plain soy yogurt and half organic banana, sliced, and a sprinkle of granola.

Christopher's Crazy Crepes

Makes 12 to 16 crepes

1 cup whole wheat pastry flour
Pinch of salt
1¼ cups soy or rice milk
2 cage-free eggs
2 tablespoons soy margarine,
   melted and cooled
2 to 3 tablespoons margarine

Combine flour, salt, and soy milk in a large bowl. Beat until smooth. Beat the eggs in a small bowl and stir in the melted margarine. Add to the flour and soy milk mixture and beat until smooth. For best results, refrigerate for 1 hour and beat again.

Place a small nonstick skillet with shallow sides over medium heat. When a drop of water skitters across the skillet, add ½ teaspoon of the margarine. Put about 1 tablespoon of batter into the skillet and swirl it around so it forms a thin layer on the bottom of the pan. Pour out the excess. It will cook in less than 1 minute. When the batter appears dry, flip and cook about 15 more seconds. The crepe should not become crisp at all. Repeat the process, each time adding margarine to the skillet.

The crepes can be filled with a fruit jam or any peeled and seeded fruit and a little maple sugar cooked briefly. Place on an ovenproof platter and heat in the oven, if desired.

Flavorful French Toast

Makes 4 servings

2 cage-free eggs
¾ cup vanilla soy or rice milk
1 teaspoon ground cinnamon
½ tablespoon maple sugar (optional)
Canola oil or soy margarine, as needed
4 slices whole grain bread

Preheat a large skillet over medium heat. In a wide bowl, beat the eggs. Add the soy milk, cinnamon, and maple sugar. Beat a little more.

Add about 1 tablespoon margarine or oil to the skillet. When it is hot, soak each side of a slice of bread and place on the griddle. Cook until nicely browned, about 2 minutes. For a little more fun, after dipping in the egg mixture, coat with crushed cornflakes and cook as usual.

Honey-Cinnamon Toast

Makes 1 serving

2 slices whole grain bread
1½ to 2 teaspoons soy margarine
    for spreading
1 to 1½ teaspoons honey
½ teaspoon ground cinnamon

Toast the bread. Spread half the margarine on each slice, then half the honey, and sprinkle with half the cinnamon.

Double Delicious

Makes 1 sandwich

2 slices whole wheat bread

1 tablespoon soy cream cheese

All-natural strawberry jam for spreading,
   plus extra for garnish

1 cage-free egg

1 teaspoon soy milk

1 tablespoon soy margarine

Make a sandwich with the bread, cream cheese, and jam. In a shallow bowl, beat the egg and soy milk. Dip the sandwich in egg, soaking both sides.

Put the soy margarine in a frying pan. Add the sandwich and fry until golden brown, about 2 minutes per side. Serve with a spoonful of jam on top.

Breakfast Biscuits

Makes 12 biscuits

2 cups whole wheat pastry flour
   or unbleached flour

½ teaspoon baking soda

2 teaspoons baking powder

½ teaspoon salt

6 tablespoons soy margarine

1 cup soy cream

Preheat the oven to 450 degrees. Grease a sheet pan.

In a large bowl, stir the flour, baking soda, baking powder, and salt. Cut in the margarine with 2 knives until the mixture looks like coarse cornmeal. Pour in the soy cream and stir with a fork until the dry ingredients are evenly moistened.

Lightly flour a work surface. Turn out the dough and pat into a circle about ¾ inch thick. Cut into rounds with a glass. Put on the sheet pan and bake about 15 to 20 minutes, until lightly browned.

Oatmeal

Serves 4

2½ cups water
1½ cups rolled oats
2 tablespoons maple syrup, plus
   additional for drizzling
1½ tablespoons raisins
1 teaspoon ground cinnamon
½ organic banana, sliced (optional)

Bring the water to a boil in a medium pot. Add the oats and stir. Cook 5 minutes over medium heat. Remove from the heat and add the maple syrup, raisins, and cinnamon. Put in a bowl. Drizzle with maple syrup, and top with fresh banana slices if desired.

Oatmeal Banana Blast

Serves 4

2½ cups water
1½ cups rolled oats
1 tablespoon organic mashed banana
1 tablespoon vanilla soy yogurt
1 drop vanilla extract

Bring the water to a boil in a medium pot and add the oats. Cook 5 minutes, stirring occasionally. Put in a bowl and stir in the mashed banana, soy yogurt, and vanilla.

Cornmeal Cereal

Serves 2

2 cups water
2 cups vanilla soy or rice milk
1 cup fine white or yellow cornmeal
Salt to taste
1 teaspoon vanilla
Soy margarine to taste
Unsulfured molasses for sweetening

Bring the water and soy milk to a light boil in a medium pot. Gradually whisk in the cornmeal. Add a few pinches of salt and lower the heat. Cook until thickened, stirring frequently. Fine cornmeal will be done in 4 to 5 minutes, coarse grits in 30 to 40 minutes. When done, stir in the vanilla and margarine to taste. Serve with molasses.

Maple-Nut Cereal

Serves 2

2 cups water
2 cups vanilla soy milk or rice milk,
    plus extra for serving
Salt
1 cup Cream of Wheat
½ teaspoon ground cinnamon
½ cup toasted pecans
Maple syrup for sweetening

In a medium pot, mix the water and soy milk together and bring to a boil. Stir in the salt, cereal, and cinnamon. Continue stirring for a few minutes, lower the heat, and cover. Cook about 7 minutes, until thick. Pour into 2 bowls, sprinkle nuts on top, and drizzle with maple syrup. Add a little soy milk and serve.

Granola

Makes 9 cups

3 cups rolled oats

⅓ cup unprocessed coarse bran

½ cup raw sunflower seeds

¼ cup honey

¼ cup maple syrup

½ cup cashews

½ cup pecans

¼ cup peanuts

¼ teaspoon ground allspice

¼ teaspoon ground cinnamon

2 cups mixed dried fruit, such as raisins,
     chopped apricots, and berries

½ cup toasted wheat germ

Preheat the oven to 350 degrees. Spread the oats, bran, and seeds on a jelly-roll pan and bake for 15 minutes, until golden brown.

Put the honey, maple syrup, nuts, and spices in a large bowl. When the oats are done, stir them into the honey mixture. Return the mixture to the pan, spreading it out evenly. Toast in the oven for 10 minutes, stirring occasionally, until it's evenly browned. Toss the mixture with the dried fruit and wheat germ. Cool completely.

VARIATION

For breakfast sundaes, fill parfait glasses with fresh peaches and berries. Add plain soy yogurt and top with granola.

Breakfast Burrito

Serves 4

6 cage-free eggs, beaten
Six 8-inch whole wheat tortillas
1 tablespoon soy margarine
½ cup grated white soy cheese
1 organic plum tomato
½ organic avocado, diced
Salsa (optional)

Preheat the oven to 250 degrees. Beat the eggs in a medium bowl. Warm the tortillas on a rack. Meanwhile, in a large nonstick pan over medium-high heat, melt the margarine. Scramble and cook the eggs. Fill the tortillas with the eggs and remaining ingredients and fold into burritos.

Soft-Boiled Cage-Free Eggs

Boil water in a pot. Use a pin or needle to poke a hole in the wider end of each egg. Place each egg on a spoon and gently lower it into the boiling water. Cook 3 to 4 minutes. Run each egg under cold water briefly. Crack the eggshell, and scoop the egg out.

VARIATIONS

Medium-Boiled Eggs: Increase the boiling time to 5 or 6 minutes, and hold the cooked egg under cold running water for 30 seconds. Crack and peel.

Hard-Boiled Eggs: Increase the boiling time to 12 to 15 minutes. Hold under cold running water for 30 seconds. Crack and peel.

Basic Omelette

Serves 2

4 to 5 cage-free eggs
2 tablespoons plain soy milk
Spike or salt and pepper to taste
2 tablespoons soy margarine or olive oil

In a bowl, beat the eggs and soy milk until blended. Add the Spike or salt and pepper to taste. In a medium to large skillet, heat the margarine or olive oil over medium-high heat. When the margarine has melted, swirl it around in the pan. Pour in the egg mixture. Cook undisturbed for about 30 seconds. With a spatula, push the edges of the eggs to the center of the pan. Cook about 3 minutes, until the eggs are no longer runny. Add your choice of omelette fillings. With a large spatula, flip half of the omelette over and put on a serving platter.

FILLINGS

Grated soy cheese

Organic avocado, organic tomato, soy sour cream

Organic mushrooms: Before making the omelette, sauté 1 cup mushrooms in 2 teaspoons olive oil or soy margarine. Season with Spike or salt and pepper and freshly pressed garlic. Add to the omelette.

Herbs: Finely chop 2 tablespoons parsley, 1 tablespoon marjoram, and ½ teaspoon chervil. Whisk the herbs directly into the beaten eggs.

Soy ham and cheese: Before making the omelette, sauté 2 pieces sliced soy ham in 1 tablespoon olive oil for 3 to 4 minutes, until browned. Add ¼ cup grated soy cheese just before folding the omelette.

Organic apples: Peel and grate 1 apple. Sauté lightly in ½ teaspoon soy margarine. Add 1 teaspoon maple sugar and ½ teaspoon ground cinnamon. Serve with the omelette.

Eggs in a Hole

Makes 1 to 2 servings

2 slices whole grain bread
1 teaspoon to 1 tablespoon soy margarine
2 cage-free eggs
Salt and pepper or Spike to taste

Take a small glass and place on top of a bread slice; press, then remove the round piece. (Or take a cookie cutter and do the same; make a heart or star, if you like.) Do the same with the remaining slice of bread.

Heat a medium nonstick skillet over medium heat for about 1 minute. Add margarine to coat the skillet. Place a slice of bread in the pan. Crack 1 egg directly into the hole. Cook until the white is no longer translucent, about 1 minute. Flip and cook about 1 minute more. Season it with salt and pepper. Cook the remaining slice of bread and egg. Toast the little rounds and place, with margarine and jam, on the side.

Gabby's Gourmet Cheese and Eggs

Makes 2 servings

1 tablespoon soy margarine
4 cage-free eggs
Salt and pepper or Spike to taste
1 to 2 tablespoons soy cream or soy milk
½ cup grated soy cheese

Melt the margarine in a medium skillet over medium heat. Beat the eggs in a medium bowl. Add salt, pepper, and soy cream. Add the egg mixture to the skillet and lower the heat to medium-low. Add the soy cheese and stir frequently for 2 to 4 minutes, until the eggs reach the desired consistency.

Hash Browns

Serves 6

1 to 1½ pounds organic russet potatoes, peeled
3 tablespoons soy margarine or olive oil
Salt and pepper or Spike to taste

In a medium saucepan, cover the potatoes with cold water. Bring to a boil. Cook until just about tender. Let cool. Then grate the potatoes.

Heat the margarine or olive oil in a large skillet. Add the potatoes, salt, and pepper. Flatten the potatoes with a spatula. Cook about 5 minutes, until golden brown. Flip and brown the other side. Serve.

Breakfast Fruit Salad

Serves 4

¼ cup unsweetened coconut
1 cup chopped organic pineapple
1 cup chopped organic mango
1 cup chopped organic orange
1 cup sliced organic banana
¼ cup honey

Toast the coconut. Toss the fruits together with the honey in a serving bowl. Sprinkle the coconut on top. Serve as a side dish or on its own.

MUFFINS

Blueberry Muffins

Makes 18 muffins

2 cups unbleached flour

⅔ cup Sucanat

2½ teaspoons baking powder

¼ teaspoon baking soda

½ teaspoon salt

1 teaspoon ground cinnamon

1 cup soy milk

½ cup soy margarine, melted

2 cage-free eggs

1 cup organic blueberries

Preheat the oven to 400 degrees. Grease the muffin tins.

In a medium bowl, mix the dry ingredients. Set aside. In a large bowl, whisk together the soy milk, margarine, and eggs until smooth. Add the dry ingredients and stir until well blended. Add the berries and stir until well incorporated.

Spoon the batter into the muffin cups, and bake 15 to 20 minutes. The muffins are done when a toothpick inserted in the center comes out clean. Cool 5 minutes in the tins, then remove.

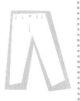

Mary Ann's Rappin' Raspberry Muffins

Makes 18 muffins

2 cups unbleached flour
2 teaspoons baking powder
1 teaspoon baking soda
½ teaspoon salt
⅔ cup Sucanat
½ cup soy margarine, melted
2 cage-free eggs
½ cup soy milk
1 teaspoon grated lemon zest
½ teaspoon almond extract
1 cup organic raspberries

Preheat the oven to 375 degrees. Grease the muffin tins.

In a large bowl, stir together the flour, baking powder, baking soda, salt, and Sucanat. In a medium bowl, combine the margarine, eggs, soy milk, lemon zest, and almond extract. Add to the dry ingredients. Stir just until blended, fold in the raspberries, and spoon the batter into muffin cups. Bake about 20 minutes, or until a toothpick inserted in the center of a muffin comes out clean. Cool in the tins 5 minutes and remove.

Apple-Cinnamon Muffins

Makes 1 dozen muffins

1 cup quick-cooking rolled oats
1 cup soy milk
1 organic apple
1 cage-free egg
⅓ cup date or maple sugar
⅓ cup cooking oil
1 cup unbleached flour or whole wheat flour
1 teaspoon baking powder
½ teaspoon baking soda
½ teaspoon salt
1½ teaspoons ground cinnamon
2 tablespoons maple sugar

Preheat the oven to 400 degrees. Grease the muffin tins.

Put the oats and soy milk in a medium bowl. Stir and set aside. Peel, core, and chop the apple into small pieces. In the bowl of an electric mixer, combine the egg, date or maple sugar, and oil. Mix on low until smooth. Add the oat and soy milk mixture to this and beat until blended. Add the flour, baking powder, baking soda, salt, and ½ teaspoon of the cinnamon. With a wooden spoon, mix all the ingredients until well blended. Do not overblend. Add the apples and stir.

Fill 12 muffin cups about two-thirds full and set aside. In a small bowl, mix the 2 tablespoons maple sugar and remaining 1 teaspoon cinnamon. Sprinkle over the muffins. Bake 20 to 25 minutes, until a toothpick inserted in the center of a muffin comes out clean. Cool in the tins 5 minutes and remove.

O's Banana-Oat Muffins

Makes 1 dozen muffins

1½ cups whole wheat pastry flour

1 teaspoon grated nutmeg

1½ teaspoons baking soda

2 large, ripe, organic bananas, mashed

¾ cup soy milk

⅓ cup maple sugar

1 cage-free egg

2 tablespoons soy margarine, melted

1 cup rolled oats

Preheat the oven to 375 degrees. Grease the muffin tins.

In a medium bowl, mix the flour, nutmeg, and baking soda. In a large bowl, mix the bananas, soy milk, maple sugar, egg, and margarine. Add the oats. Stir in the flour mixture. Fill the muffin cups two-thirds full and bake for about 25 minutes, until a toothpick inserted in the center of a muffin comes out clean. Cool in the tins 5 minutes, then remove.

Buckwheat Kasha Bread

Yields 1 loaf

¼ cup kasha

⅓ cup boiling water

1 cup buckwheat flour

1 cup unbleached flour

½ cup maple or date sugar

1 teaspoon baking powder

1 teaspoon baking soda

½ teaspoon salt

1 cup soy cream

1 cage-free egg

¼ cup cooking oil

½ cup chopped walnuts

In a small bowl, mix the kasha and boiling water. Let sit 15 minutes. Preheat the oven to 350 degrees. Grease and flour a medium loaf pan.

In a large bowl, mix the buckwheat flour, unbleached flour, maple or date sugar, baking powder, baking soda, and salt. Set aside. In a small bowl, whisk together the soy cream, egg, and oil until smooth. Stir in the nuts and kasha. Add the wet ingredients to the dry ingredients and stir until just blended. Spread evenly in the prepared pan. Bake for about 1 hour, until a thin wooden skewer inserted in the center of the loaf comes out clean. Cool in the pan for 10 minutes. Remove and place on wire racks to finish cooling.

Parker's Poppy Seed Muffins

Makes 1 dozen

1½ cups unbleached flour
½ cup toasted wheat germ
⅓ cup poppy seeds
⅓ cup Sucanat
1 tablespoon baking powder
½ teaspoon salt
1 cup soy milk
1 cage-free egg
¼ cup soy margarine, melted

Preheat the oven to 400 degrees. Grease the muffin tins.

In a large bowl, stir together the flour, wheat germ, poppy seeds, Sucanat, baking powder, and salt. In a small bowl, whisk together the soy milk, egg, and margarine until smooth. Add to the dry ingredients and stir until blended.

Spoon the batter into the muffin cups. Bake 15 to 18 minutes, or until a toothpick inserted in the center of a muffin comes out clean. Cool for 5 minutes in the tins and remove.

Banana Nut Bread

Makes 2 loaves

2½ cups whole wheat flour

2 teaspoons baking soda

1 teaspoon salt

1 cup soy margarine

2 cups date sugar or Sucanat

2 cups ripe organic bananas

4 cage-free eggs

1 cup chopped pecans or walnuts

Preheat the oven to 350 degrees. Grease and flour two 8½-inch loaf pans.

In a medium bowl, stir the flour, baking soda, and salt and set aside. In a large bowl, beat the margarine and sugar until blended. Beat in the banana and then the eggs, stirring until well mixed. Add the dry ingredients and stir until blended. Divide the batter evenly between the 2 pans and bake until a thin wooden skewer inserted in the center of a loaf comes out clean, 55 to 65 minutes. Cool the loaves in the pans for 10 minutes. Remove and place on wire racks to finish cooling.

Pumpkin Muffins

Makes 2 dozen muffins

3½ cups unbleached flour

1 tablespoon baking powder

2 teaspoons pumpkin pie spice

1 teaspoon baking soda

1 teaspoon salt

3 large cage-free eggs

1 can (16 ounces) pumpkin

¾ cup soy margarine, melted

⅔ cup maple sugar

⅔ cup honey

⅔ cup soy milk

1 teaspoon ground cinnamon

Preheat the oven to 400 degrees. Grease the muffin tins.

In a large bowl, mix the flour, baking powder, pumpkin spice, baking soda, and salt. In a medium bowl, whisk the eggs, pumpkin, melted soy margarine, maple sugar, honey, soy milk, and cinnamon. Add the wet ingredients to the dry ingredients and combine well.

Spoon the batter into the muffin tins and bake for 25 to 30 minutes, until a toothpick inserted in the center of a muffin comes out clean. Cool in the pan 5 minutes and remove.

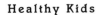

Joey's Jammin' Peanut Butter and Jelly Muffins

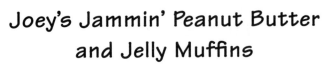

Makes 1 dozen muffins

1¾ cups unbleached flour

⅓ cup Sucanat

2½ teaspoons baking powder

½ teaspoon salt

½ cup creamy peanut butter

1 large cage-free egg

¾ cup soy milk

⅓ cup soy margarine, melted

½ cup jam of choice

Preheat the oven to 375 degrees. Grease the muffin tins.

In a large bowl, mix the flour, Sucanat, baking powder, and salt. In another bowl, beat the peanut butter and egg, and add the soy milk, stirring, a little at a time. Add the margarine and mix well. Combine the wet and dry ingredients and stir. The batter will become stiff.

Put 1 heaping tablespoon of batter in each muffin cup. Use your finger to make a well in each one. Put 1 teaspoon of jam in each hole. Cover with another heaping tablespoon of batter. Spread the batter on top gently so no jam is visible. Bake 20 minutes, or until a toothpick inserted in the center of a muffin comes out clean. Cool in the tins for 5 minutes and remove.

Peanut Butter and Chocolate Chip Muffins

Makes 1 dozen muffins

2 cups unbleached flour

⅓ cup Sucanat

1 tablespoon baking powder

½ teaspoon salt

⅔ cup creamy all-natural peanut butter

1⅓ cups soy milk

¼ cup soy margarine, melted

2 cage-free eggs

½ cup chopped roasted peanuts

1 cup grain-sweetened chocolate chips

Preheat the oven to 400 degrees. Grease the muffin tins.

In a large bowl, stir together the flour, Sucanat, baking powder, and salt. In a medium bowl, beat the peanut butter until smooth; then beat in a few spoonfuls of the soy milk. Beat in the rest of the soy milk, then beat in the margarine and eggs. Stir in the peanuts and chocolate chips. Add the wet ingredients to the dry ingredients and stir until blended.

Spoon the batter into the muffin cups. Bake about 15 minutes, or until a toothpick inserted in the center of a muffin comes out clean. Cool 5 minutes in the tins and remove.

S M O O T H I E S

Banana Smoothie

Serves 1

1 organic banana
¾ cup vanilla soy milk
¼ cup plain soy yogurt
1 teaspoon honey
8 ice cubes

Put all the ingredients into a blender and blend until smooth.

Blueberry-Banana Smoothie

Serves 1

1½ cups vanilla soy milk
1 cup organic frozen blueberries
1 cup organic banana
1 tablespoon honey
2 tablespoons protein powder
4 to 6 ice cubes

Put all the ingredients into a blender and blend until smooth.

Banana-Berry Smoothie

Serves 1

1½ cups vanilla soy milk
½ cup frozen organic banana
½ cup frozen organic strawberries
½ cup frozen organic raspberries
¼ cup frozen organic blueberries
2 tablespoons protein powder
2 to 4 ice cubes

Put all the ingredients into a blender and blend until smooth.

Strawberry-Banana Smoothie

Serves 1

1½ cups vanilla soy milk
2 tablespoons protein powder
½ cup sliced organic banana
½ cup frozen organic strawberries
1 tablespoon honey
6 to 8 ice cubes

Put all the ingredients into a blender and blend until smooth.

Orange Nut Smoothie

Serves 1

1 cup organic orange juice

1 cup soy milk

1 organic frozen banana

2 tablespoons almond butter

6 ice cubes

Put all the ingredients into a blender and blend until smooth.

Brilliant Blueberry-Peach Smoothie

Serves 1

1½ cups vanilla soy milk

1 cup frozen organic peaches

1 cup frozen organic blueberries

1 tablespoon honey

4 to 6 ice cubes

Put all the ingredients into a blender and blend until smooth.

Mango-Peach Smoothie

Serves 1

1 cup organic frozen peaches

1 cup organic frozen mango

1½ cups vanilla soy milk

1 tablespoon honey

Put all the ingredients into a blender and blend until smooth.

Mango-Date Smoothie

Serves 1

1½ cups vanilla soy milk

1 cup organic frozen mango

1 cup organic frozen papaya

½ cup vanilla or plain soy yogurt

½ cup chopped dates

2 tablespoons protein powder

4 to 6 ice cubes

Put all the ingredients into a blender and blend until smooth.

Nutty Nicky's Honey Nut Smoothie

Serves 1

1 cup vanilla soy milk

1 cup vanilla soy yogurt

1 frozen organic banana

2 tablespoons protein powder

3 tablespoons almond butter

1 tablespoon honey

1 teaspoon almond extract

4 to 6 ice cubes

Put all the ingredients into a blender and blend until smooth.

225

Gabbin' Gabby's Granola Smoothie

Serves 1

1½ cups vanilla soy milk

½ cup granola

½ cup vanilla soy yogurt

1 organic frozen banana

4 to 6 ice cubes

Put all the ingredients into a blender and blend until smooth.

Lynn's Super Smoothie

Serves 1

1 organic banana

1 cup organic mixed berries, such as
blackberries and blueberries

1 cup vanilla soy or rice milk

1 cup vanilla soy yogurt

1 scoop vanilla soy protein powder

1 heaping teaspoon psyllium husks

1 tablespoon ground flaxseeds

1 tablespoon flaxseed oil

2 capsules acidophilus

1 pinch alfalfa

Put all the ingredients into a blender and blend until smooth.

S N A C K S

Currant Scones

Serves 10

2 cups unbleached flour
¼ cup Sucanat
1 teaspoon cream of tartar
1 teaspoon baking soda
½ teaspoon salt
½ cup soy margarine
⅔ to ¾ cup soy milk
¾ cup dried currants

Preheat the oven to 400 degrees. Mix the flour, Sucanat, cream of tartar, baking soda, and salt in a large bowl. Add the margarine and stir until the mixture resembles coarse cornmeal. Gradually add the soy milk to make a soft dough. Add the currants and knead the dough 3 or 4 times.

On a lightly floured surface, roll out the dough to ½ inch thickness and cut out the scones with a 2-inch cookie cutter. Place on an ungreased cookie sheet. Bake 10 to 12 minutes.

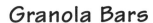
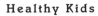

Granola Bars

¾ cup creamy all-natural peanut butter

½ cup plus 2 tablespoons honey

2 cups granola

1 cup rolled oats

¾ cup raisins

¾ cup chopped dried organic apricots

½ cup dried organic cranberries

½ cup sunflower seeds

½ cup peanuts

2 cage-free eggs, lightly beaten

2 cups crispy rice cereal (a health food brand)

Preheat the oven to 325 degrees. Grease a 13-by-9-by-2-inch baking pan.

In a small pan over low heat, melt the peanut butter and honey. Let the mixture cool.

In a large bowl, mix the granola, oats, raisins, apricots, cranberries, sunflower seeds, and peanuts. Stir in the peanut butter mixture, making sure that everything is coated. Mix in the eggs slowly. Gently stir in the rice cereal and press the mixture into the prepared pan to form an even layer. Bake for 20 to 30 minutes, until lightly browned on the edges. Cool in the pan and cut into squares.

Very Nice Cinnamon and Spice Applesauce

Serves 4

6 medium organic apples
2 tablespoons fresh lemon juice
½ cup purified water
⅓ cup Sucanat or maple sugar
½ teaspoon ground cinnamon
½ teaspoon ground cloves

Peel, core, and chop the apples into small pieces. Put the pieces into a large saucepan, and sprinkle with the lemon juice. Add the remaining ingredients. Bring to a boil over medium heat, stirring occasionally with a wooden spoon. Reduce the heat and cover the pan. Simmer for 20 to 30 minutes, until the apples are mushy. Add more water if necessary to keep the apples from sticking. Remove from the heat and let cool for 15 minutes. When the apples have cooled a little, mash them until you get the texture you want, thick or smooth.

Sydney's Simply Super Fruit Salad

Serves 4

½ cup plain soy yogurt

2 tablespoons Nayonnaise

1½ tablespoons maple syrup

4 large organic lettuce leaves

2 medium organic plums

1 large organic apple

1 medium organic pear

⅔ cup seedless organic red grapes

2 tablespoons chopped walnuts

Ground cinnamon to taste

To make the sauce, in a small bowl, use a spoon to blend the soy yogurt, Nayonnaise, and maple syrup. Set aside.

Line each of 4 small bowls with a lettuce leaf and set aside.

Cut each plum in half, remove the pit, and cut each half into 6 pieces. Cut the apple and pear into quarters and remove the stems and seeds. Cut each quarter into 4 pieces. Put equal amounts of fruit in each serving dish. Toss and top the fruit with the soy yogurt sauce. Sprinkle each with ½ tablespoon walnuts. Sprinkle with cinnamon and serve.

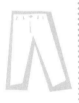

Edamame

2 tablespoons salt

1 pound frozen organic edamame (soybeans)

Fill half to three-quarters of a medium pot with water and bring to a boil. Add the salt and edamame and return to a boil. Cook 5 minutes. Drain and rinse with cold water.

Guacamole

Serves 4 to 6

3 large ripe organic avocados,
   mashed (reserve 1 pit)
1 organic tomato, chopped
½ large organic red onion,
   finely chopped
½ cup fresh chopped cilantro
½ teaspoon Spike
1½ tablespoons fresh lime juice

Mix all the ingredients in a bowl. Place the avocado pit in the middle to prevent discoloration. Cover and refrigerate.

Salsa

Serves 4 to 6

2½ to 3 pounds ripe organic tomatoes
1 white onion, peeled and chopped
½ cup fresh chopped cilantro
½ to 1 teaspoon salt
2 tablespoons fresh lime juice

Combine all the ingredients in a bowl. Cover and refrigerate.

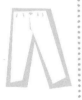

S O U P S

Gazpacho

Serves 6 to 8

2 organic cucumbers,
    peeled, seeded, and diced
3 organic beefsteak
    tomatoes, diced
4 cloves garlic, pressed
1 red onion, coarsely
    chopped
2 tablespoons olive oil

¼ cup red wine vinegar
¼ cup balsamic vinegar
3 cups organic tomato juice
1 teaspoon salt
1 teaspoon black pepper
¼ cup chopped fresh cilantro
    leaves, plus 1 leaf for
    garnish

In a large bowl, mix the cucumbers, tomatoes, garlic, onion, olive oil, vinegars, and tomato juice. Toss to combine. Put half of the mixture into a food processor or blender. Pulse 6 to 8 times until it is a slightly chunky puree. Return to the original bowl. Add the salt, pepper, and cilantro and mix. Garnish with the cilantro leaf and serve.

Garden Vegetable Soup

Serves 8

11½ cups water

4 cups chopped organic onions

3 stalks organic celery, chopped

2 cups chopped organic broccoli

1 cup chopped organic carrots

1 cup chopped organic cauliflower

2 cups chopped organic zucchini

1½ cups brown rice

1 large potato, unpeeled, diced

1 tablespoon chopped garlic

½ cup tamari sauce

¼ cup Bragg Liquid Aminos

2 tablespoons dried parsley

In a large pot, bring ½ cup of the water to a gentle boil and cook the onions and celery until soft. Add the remaining water and the rest of the ingredients and bring to a boil. Reduce the heat to medium, cover, and cook for 1 hour. Uncover and cook 30 minutes more.

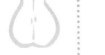

Pumpkin Soup

Serves 6

1 can (16 ounces) organic
   pumpkin
3 organic carrots, sliced
3 organic celery stalks, sliced
1 organic onion, chopped
1 bay leaf

6 cups vegetable broth
1 cup soy cream
½ teaspoon ground nutmeg
1 tablespoon honey
Salt and pepper to taste

Place the pumpkin, carrots, celery, onion, bay leaf, and broth in a large pot and bring to a boil. Lower the heat, cover, and simmer about 30 minutes. Remove from the heat and put the mixture in a food processor or blender. Puree and return to the pot. Stir in the remaining ingredients. Add extra soy cream for a thicker consistency, if desired.

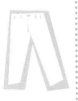

Lentil Soup

Serves 8

14½ cups water
2 cups chopped organic
   onions
2 organic celery stalks,
   chopped
1½ cups sliced organic
   carrots
1½ cups chopped organic
   broccoli

1½ cups chopped potatoes
3 cups dried lentils, rinsed
½ teaspoon cumin
⅓ cup Bragg Liquid Aminos
⅓ cup tamari sauce
Salt and pepper to taste

In a large pot, bring ½ cup of the water to a gentle boil and cook the onions and celery until soft. Add the remaining 14 cups water and the rest of the ingredients. Bring to a boil, reduce the heat to medium, and cook 1½ hours.

Split Pea Soup

Serves 8

15½ cups water
3½ cups chopped onions
1½ organic celery stalks, chopped
2 cups chopped organic broccoli
4 cups dried split peas, rinsed
1 teaspoon salt or Spike
1 tablespoon chopped garlic
2 tablespoons tamari sauce
½ teaspoon dried thyme
½ cup brown rice

In a large pot, bring ½ cup of the water to a gentle boil and cook the onions until soft. Add the remaining 15 cups water and the rest of the ingredients. Return to a boil. Lower the heat to medium, and cook 1½ hours.

Little Ole Sweet Pea Soup

Serves 8

10 cups water

3¼ cups dried green split peas, rinsed

1½ cups diced organic white onion

2 cups diced unpeeled organic yam

2½ cups chopped organic celery

¼ cup olive oil

1 pound organic spinach, trimmed,
    rinsed, drained, and chopped

1 tablespoon crumbled basil leaves

One 10-ounce package frozen organic
    peas, thawed

3 tablespoons Bragg Liquid Aminos

3 tablespoons light molasses

2 teaspoons Spike

In a 6- to 8-quart pot, combine the water, split peas, onion, yam, celery, and olive oil. Bring to a boil, reduce the heat, and simmer, covered, for about 30 minutes. Add the spinach and basil and return to a boil. Reduce the heat and simmer, covered, 25 to 35 minutes, stirring occasionally, until the peas have dissolved into a thick broth. Add the frozen peas, Bragg's, molasses, and Spike. Simmer 5 more minutes, and serve.

Lucky Lima Bean Soup

Serves 6

10½ cups water

1½ cups chopped organic onions

¼ cup vegetable stock

1 cup chopped organic celery

2 cups sliced organic carrots

2 cups chopped organic yams

1 cup chopped organic broccoli

1 teaspoon minced basil

1½ cups dried baby lima beans, rinsed

¾ cup Bragg's liquid aminos

½ teaspoon dried parsley

In a large pot, bring ½ cup of the water to a gentle boil and cook the onions until they are soft. Add the remaining 10 cups water and the rest of the ingredients. Bring to a boil, then lower the heat to medium. Cook, uncovered, until the lima beans are soft, about 1½ to 2½ hours.

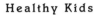

Madison's Minestrone

Serves 8

1 medium organic onion, chopped

1 large organic carrot, unpeeled and chopped

1 organic celery stalk, chopped

1 tablespoon olive oil

2 Italian-style turkey sausages or soy sausages, peeled

4 cups vegetable or chicken broth

1 medium organic zucchini, chopped

⅓ cup broken spaghetti (1-inch pieces)

½ teaspoon dried oregano

1 can (28 ounces) crushed organic tomatoes

Salt and pepper or Spike to taste

Soy Parmesan for sprinkling

Put the onion, carrot, celery, oil, and sausages into a large saucepan over medium heat. Cook until sausages loses all of its pink color, about 5 to 10 minutes. Add the broth, zucchini, spaghetti pieces, oregano, and tomatoes and stir. Bring to a boil, reduce the heat to low, and simmer, uncovered, about 30 minutes. Season with salt and pepper. Serve with a little soy Parmesan on top.

Rose's Macaroni Soup

Serves 6

2¼ teaspoons salt

3 cups macaroni (elbow or shell)

1 medium organic onion

½ large free-range chicken

2 bay leaves

1 teaspoon soy margarine

¼ teaspoon black pepper

1 large organic carrot, cut into
    ¼-inch pieces

¾ cup soy milk

Bring a large pot of water to a boil, add ¼ teaspoon of the salt, and cook the macaroni until al dente. Rinse with cold water and set aside. Cut the onion in half and chop one of the halves. Set the chopped onion aside.

Put the chicken in a medium pot, add enough water to cover, the ½ onion (not the chopped), bay leaves, and remaining 2 teaspoons salt. Bring to a boil. Lower the heat to medium and simmer for 20 minutes, or until the chicken is cooked. (Do not overcook the chicken.) Take out the chicken and let cool. Cut the white meat into ½-inch pieces. (Reserve the dark meat for another use.) Strain the soup, pour the broth back in the pot, and bring to a boil over very low heat.

Melt the margarine in a medium skillet over medium heat and sauté the chopped onion until translucent. Add the cut-up chicken and black pepper. Sauté for 3 minutes (do not let the onion brown). Add to the soup pot. Make sure that there are 6 cups of broth. If not, add water or packaged broth. Raise the heat to high. Add the carrot and boil for 5 minutes. Add the macaroni and soy milk, and stir. Enjoy it while it's hot.

SIDE DISHES

Green Salad

Serves 6 to 8

6 handfuls organic salad
    greens
½ organic avocado, coarsely
    chopped
½ cup sliced organic
    cucumber
8 organic cherry tomatoes,
    halved

¼ cup sunflower seeds
1 clove garlic, pressed
1 teaspoon Spike
1 cup organic tahini
1 teaspoon ground cumin
¼ cup fresh lemon juice
½ cup water

In a large bowl, combine the salad greens, avocado, cucumber, cherry tomatoes, and sunflower seeds.

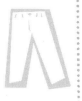

Put the garlic, Spike, tahini, cumin, and lemon juice into a food processor or blender. Add the water, bit by bit, processing continuously, until the dressing reaches the proper consistency. Pour onto the mixed greens, toss, and serve.

Easy Caesar

Serves 4

⅓ cup olive oil

Juice of ½ organic lemon

6 to 8 anchovy fillets

1 clove garlic

1 large head organic romaine lettuce,
  leaves separated, rinsed, and drained

¼ cup plus 2 tablespoons soy Parmesan

1 cup whole grain dairy-free croutons

In a blender or food processor, put the oil, lemon juice, anchovies, and garlic. Blend until smooth.

Tear the lettuce into bite-sized pieces and put in a salad bowl. Sprinkle with soy Parmesan, pour the dressing over the lettuce, and toss. Top with croutons.

Tomato and Basil with Soy Mozzarella

Serves 8

6 large ripe organic tomatoes, sliced thick

1 pound soy mozzarella, sliced thick

1 bunch fresh basil, rinsed, dried, and minced

¼ cup olive oil

Salt and pepper to taste

Alternate tomato and cheese slices on a large serving platter. Sprinkle with basil and drizzle with olive oil. Salt and pepper lightly.

Healthy Waldorf Salad

Serves 6

2½ cups chopped organic apple
1 cup soy cheddar cheese chunks
1 cup organic red grapes
½ cup diced organic celery
½ cup walnut pieces
½ cup raisins
⅓ cup Nayonnaise
1 tablespoon fresh organic lemon juice

Toss all the ingredients in a large bowl, making sure to coat everything with the Nayonnaise. Refrigerate until ready to serve.

Coleslaw

Serves 6 to 8

½ cup Nayonnaise
1 teaspoon soy milk
1 tablespoon vinegar
½ teaspoon Sucanat
¼ teaspoon salt
⅛ teaspoon paprika

⅛ teaspoon pepper
1 medium head organic
  cabbage
1 large organic celery stalk
1 large organic carrot
2 tablespoons minced onion

Mix the Nayonnaise with the soy milk, vinegar, Sucanat, salt, paprika, and pepper to make a dressing. Whisk and set aside.

With a sharp knife, core and shred the cabbage. Cut the celery into ¼-inch dice. Grate the carrot.

In a large bowl, toss the cabbage, celery, carrot, onion, and the dressing. Cover and refrigerate.

Potato Salad

Serves 6 to 8

Salt
1½ pounds organic red new potatoes
½ cup minced fresh parsley
¼ cup minced organic red onion
½ teaspoon dried thyme
½ to ¾ cup Nayonnaise
Pepper to taste

Bring a medium pot of water to a boil and salt it. In the meantime, peel and chop the potatoes into bite-sized pieces. Put the potatoes in the boiling water and cook for about 15 minutes, until tender but still firm. Drain. Toss the potatoes with the parsley, onion, and thyme. Add enough Nayonnaise so that the potato salad is creamy. Add salt and pepper to your taste.

Baked Beans

Serves 4

1 pound dried navy beans,
   soaked in water to cover
   for at least 2 hours
Salt
½ cup molasses

2 teaspoons dry mustard
½ cup organic sugar-free
   ketchup
1 organic onion, thinly sliced
Pepper to taste

Fill a large pot with water. Add the beans and 2 teaspoons salt, and cover. Turn the heat to high and bring to a boil; then lower the heat to a simmer. Cover loosely and cook the beans until tender, about 1 hour, adding more water if needed.

Preheat the oven to 300 degrees. Drain the beans. Mix them in a bowl with the molasses and mustard. In a large ovenproof pot with a lid, add half of the bean mixture, half the ketchup, half onion, and salt and pepper. Repeat. Bake, uncovered, for 2½ to 3 hours, checking occasionally and being careful not to let the top burn. Add water if the beans become dry.

White Bean Salad

Serves 6 to 8

1 can (19 ounces) white beans,
    rinsed and drained
1 cup cubed organic tomatoes
½ cup diced organic red onions
½ cup minced fresh parsley
2 ounces soy mozzarella, cubed
¼ cup fresh lemon juice
3 tablespoons olive oil
1 tablespoon balsamic vinegar
1 clove garlic, minced
2 teaspoons grated lemon zest
½ teaspoon dried thyme
¼ teaspoon ground pepper

In a large bowl, gently mix the beans, tomatoes, onions, parsley, and mozzarella. In a small bowl, mix the remaining ingredients. Combine and toss.

Stir-Fried Asparagus

Serves 4

1½ pounds organic asparagus
2 tablespoons olive oil
½ teaspoon salt, or to taste

Cut the asparagus diagonally into 3-inch pieces. Heat the oil in a skillet over high heat, and add the asparagus. Stir frequently, about 3 minutes, until tender-crisp. Sprinkle with salt and serve.

Spinach with Pine Nuts

Serves 4

1 bunch fresh organic spinach,
   washed well, ends trimmed
1½ teaspoons olive oil
2 tablespoons pine nuts
2 cloves garlic, chopped
Salt to taste

Cook the spinach in a large saucepan over high heat for about 5 minutes, or until tender, stirring frequently. Put in a colander and set aside. Return the pan to medium heat and add oil when hot. Add the pine nuts and garlic, and cook until golden, about 2 minutes. Add the spinach and toss together. Cook another 2 minutes. Salt to taste and serve.

Groovin' Green Beans

Serves 4

12 ounces slender organic green beans
2 tablespoons soy margarine
1 teaspoon lite tamari or low-sodium soy sauce
1½ tablespoons fresh lemon juice
8 cups water
1 teaspoon salt

Trim the green beans. In a small saucepan over low heat, melt the soy margarine. Remove from the heat. With a wooden spoon, stir in the soy sauce and lemon juice. Set aside.

   Add the water and salt to a large saucepan and bring to a boil. Add the green beans and cook about 6 minutes. Drain the beans and put in a serving bowl. Pour the sauce over them and serve.

Asparagus with Orange Dipping Sauce

Serves 4

¾ cup water

Salt

1 pound organic asparagus, trimmed and washed

3 tablespoons organic orange juice

1 teaspoon finely grated orange rind

2 teaspoons olive oil

2 teaspoons sesame oil

Pepper to taste

Fill a saucepan with the water and add ½ teaspoon salt. Bring the water to a boil. Add the asparagus and cook until tender, about 3 to 5 minutes. Rinse under cold water and towel dry.

In a small bowl, whisk together the orange rind, olive oil, and sesame oil. Add salt and pepper to taste. Arrange the asparagus on a large plate and put the dipping sauce in the middle.

Carol's Crazy Maple Carrots

Serves 4

3 or 4 organic carrots

½ cup water

2 tablespoons maple sugar

1 tablespoon soy margarine

1 teaspoon cider vinegar

Salt and pepper to taste

Peel the carrots and slice into rounds. Put them in a medium skillet with the water. Cook, covered, for 6 to 7 minutes over medium-high heat, until the carrots are soft. Uncover and add the maple sugar, soy margarine, and cider vinegar. Turn up the heat and sauté, stirring, for 2 to 3 minutes. Season with salt and pepper.

Pureed Butternut Squash
with Ginger

Serves 4

1½ pounds organic butternut squash, peeled and diced

2 tablespoons soy margarine

1½ teaspoons minced ginger

Salt and pepper or Spike

2 teaspoons maple syrup

Place the squash in a steamer basket over boiling water and steam, covered, until tender, about 20 minutes. While the squash is still hot, place in a food processor, add the margarine and ginger, and process until smooth. Transfer to a serving dish and add salt, pepper, and maple syrup.

Acorn Squash

Serves 4

1 large organic acorn squash, seeded and
    cut into 8 pieces, skin left on

1 cup vegetable broth

1 tablespoon soy margarine

1 clove garlic, pressed

1½ teaspoons chopped fresh thyme

½ to ¾ teaspoon salt

2½ teaspoons honey

Put the squash and broth in a large saucepan and bring to a boil. Reduce the heat to low. Cover and cook until tender, about 20 minutes. Push the squash to one side of the pan. Add the margarine and garlic. Cook about 3 minutes. Combine the squash and garlic, sprinkle the squash mixture with the remaining ingredients, and cook, stirring occasionally, about 5 minutes more.

Brussels Sprouts

Serves 4

1 pint organic Brussels sprouts
1 tablespoon soy margarine
Juice of ½ organic lemon
½ teaspoon nutmeg

Wash the Brussels sprouts. Steam them for about 10 minutes. Melt the margarine in a small saucepan over medium-low heat. Add the lemon juice and nutmeg, and stir. Pour over the Brussels sprouts and serve.

Mary Beth's Zucchini Fritters

Serves 4

After these have drained, I place them on a cookie sheet to freeze and then fill freezer bags. That way I can take out however many I need at a moment's notice. I pop them on an ungreased cookie sheet at 250 degrees for about 10 minutes (straight from the freezer) and my unexpected company thinks I am just a whiz-bang hostess.—Mary Beth

> 2 medium zucchinis
> 1 medium onion
> 2 cage-free eggs
> ¾ to 1 cup unflavored bread crumbs
> ½ cup rice or oat milk
> Salt and pepper
> ¼ cup olive oil

Grate the zucchinis and onion into a large bowl. Stir in the eggs and bread crumbs, and slowly add enough rice milk so that the batter is the consistency of lumpy oatmeal. Season with salt and pepper. Heat the oil in a skillet over medium heat. Drop the batter by tablespoons into the hot oil. Fry until golden on each side, about 1 to 2 minutes, and drain on paper towels.

Baked Potatoes

Makes 4 servings

4 large organic baking potatoes

Preheat the oven to 400 degrees. Scrub the potatoes and pierce with a fork. Bake for 60 to 75 minutes, until tender.

VARIATION

Try using sweet potatoes instead of russet for a sweet change.

Roasted Potatoes

Serves 4

2 pounds organic new potatoes,
   unpeeled and cut into eighths
2½ tablespoons olive oil
6 to 8 cloves garlic, unpeeled
1 to 1½ teaspoons kosher salt
2½ teaspoons fresh rosemary

Preheat the oven to 425 degrees. Put the potatoes in a roasting pan and add the olive oil, garlic, and salt. Mix to coat the potatoes. Roast 35 to 45 minutes. Remove from the oven and sprinkle with rosemary.

Mish-Mashed Potatoes

Serves 4

4 large organic russet potatoes
Salt
½ cup soy cream
3 tablespoons soy margarine,
    plus more to taste

Peel the potatoes and cut into chunks. Fill a large saucepan with water. Add salt and the potatoes. Bring the water to a boil over high heat. Reduce the heat a little and cook until the potatoes are tender, about 15 to 20 minutes.

Drain the potatoes and put back in the saucepan. Turn the heat to medium for about 30 seconds to remove any excess water. Remove from the heat. Add ¼ cup of the soy cream and 2 tablespoons of the margarine to the potatoes and mash with a potato masher. Add the remaining ¼ cup soy cream and 1 tablespoon margarine. Mash until smooth and fluffy. Add more salt and margarine to taste.

Baked Fries

Serves 4

5 organic baking potatoes
⅛ cup cooking oil
Spike or salt to taste

Preheat the oven to 400 degrees. Scrub the potatoes and cut to resemble fries.

In a large bowl, toss the potatoes with the oil, using enough oil to coat all of the fries. Spread them on a nonstick jelly roll pan. Sprinkle with salt and bake about 35 to 40 minutes.

French Fries

Serves 4

5 organic baking potatoes
Cooking oil for deep-frying
Spike or salt to taste

Scrub the potatoes or peel if preferred. Cut to resemble fries. Soak in ice water and set aside.

In a large pot, heat 3 to 4 inches of oil on medium high. Drain the potatoes and dry well. Add the potatoes to the hot oil a handful at a time. Turn the heat to high and cook about 8 to 12 minutes, until the potatoes start to brown. Remove from the heat and reduce the heat to low. Drain the potatoes on paper towels to get rid of excess oil. Return the heat to high and wait a couple of minutes. Put the potatoes back in the oil to brown, stirring occasionally. Cook 3 to 5 minutes, until golden brown. Drain on paper towels and season with Spike or salt.

Brown Rice

Serves 3 to 4

1 cup brown rice, rinsed
2½ cups water or vegetable broth
   (for extra flavor)
Salt or Spike to taste
1 tablespoon soy margarine

Add all the ingredients to a medium saucepan. Bring to a boil over medium-high heat. Cover and reduce the heat to low. Cook 40 minutes, undisturbed.

Sassy Sunflower Rice

Serves 4 to 6

4 tablespoons soy margarine

1 cup brown rice

2⅔ cups vegetable broth

3 tablespoons soy Parmesan

¼ cup sunflower seed kernels

Salt to taste

In a medium saucepan put 2 tablespoons of the soy margarine and melt over medium heat. Add the rice and stir with wooden spoon. Add the vegetable broth, stir, and bring to a boil. Reduce the heat to low. Cover and simmer until all the broth is absorbed, about 40 to 50 minutes. Remove from the heat. Add the remaining 2 tablespoons of soy margarine, the soy Parmesan, sunflower seeds, and salt. Stir lightly and serve.

Macaroni and Cheese

Serves 4

8 ounces macaroni

3 tablespoons soy margarine

3 tablespoons whole wheat flour

1 teaspoon dry mustard

3½ cups soy milk

1½ cups grated soy cheddar cheese

1 teaspoon salt

½ teaspoon white pepper

¾ cup whole wheat bread crumbs

½ teaspoon oregano

½ teaspoon basil

½ teaspoon canola oil

Preheat the oven to 350 degrees. Bring a large pot of water to a boil and cook the macaroni according to the directions on the package. Rinse under cold water, drain, and set aside.

Melt the soy margarine in a large saucepan. Add the flour and mustard and cook over low heat for 2 to 3 minutes, stirring continuously. Add the milk slowly while whisking to avoid lumps. Keep cooking the sauce until thickened. Don't boil. Remove from the heat and whisk in the soy cheese. Add the salt, pepper, and macaroni, mixing until the macaroni is coated. Pour into a greased baking dish.

In a small bowl, mix together the bread crumbs, herbs, and oil. Sprinkle over the macaroni and cheese and bake for 20 minutes. The macaroni and cheese will look moist while the bread crumbs will be browned.

ENTRÉES

Peanut Butter–Banana Sandwich

Makes 1 sandwich

2 tablespoons organic peanut butter
2 slices whole grain bread
1 organic banana, sliced thin
Honey to taste

Spread the peanut butter on a slice of bread. Add the banana slices and drizzle the honey over the banana. Top with the remaining slice of bread.

Grilled Cheese and Tomato

Makes 1 sandwich

2 slices whole grain bread
2 to 3 ounces soy cheese
2 to 3 slices organic tomato
1 tablespoon soy margarine

Assemble the bread, soy cheese, and tomato into a sandwich. Into a small skillet over medium heat, add the soy margarine. When the margarine has melted, place the sandwich in the skillet. Cover the sandwich with a small, heavy pot lid. Cook for about 2 to 3 minutes, until browned. Flip and repeat on the other side.

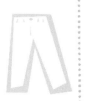

Egg Salad Sandwich

Makes 1 sandwich

6 hard-boiled cage-free eggs, chilled
2 tablespoons Nayonnaise
¼ cup chopped sweet pickle
2 tablespoons finely chopped celery
Organic lettuce leaves and tomato slices (optional)
2 slices whole grain bread

Peel the hard-boiled eggs and mash with the Nayonnaise. Mix in the pickles and celery, and spoon on a slice of bread. Add organic lettuce and tomato, if desired. Top with the remaining slice of bread.

Club Sandwich

Makes 2 sandwiches

4 slices soy bacon strips or turkey bacon
Nayonnaise
6 slices whole wheat bread, toasted
Organic lettuce leaves
8 slices soy turkey
Spike to taste
1 large organic tomato, sliced, and slices cut in half

Spray a large skillet with a little canola oil cooking spray if using soy bacon. Cook the bacon over medium heat until browned and crisp. Spread one side of each bread slice with Nayonnaise. Arrange lettuce leaves on 2 slices. Top with soy turkey and sprinkle with Spike. Cover each with another bread slice, Nayonnaise side up. Top each sandwich with more lettuce and the tomato slices. Add 2 pieces of soy bacon to each sandwich and the remaining bread, Nayonnaise side down. Cut the sandwiches diagonally into quarters. Secure each quarter with a toothpick and serve.

255

Too-Hip Tuna Sandwich

Makes 1 sandwich

1 small can of tuna
1 tablespoon Nayonnaise or canola
   oil mayonnaise, plus extra for spreading
1 tablespoon sweet relish
½ teaspoon Spike
1 leaf organic lettuce
2 slices organic tomato
2 slices whole grain bread

Drain the tuna. In a small bowl, mix it with the Nayonnaise, relish, and Spike. Lightly spread a little Nayonnaise on both slices of bread. Assemble the bread, lettuce, tomato, and a scoop of tuna into a sandwich.

VARIATION

Tuna Melt: Melt 1 tablespoon of soy margarine in a small skillet over medium heat. Assemble the tuna and 2 to 3 ounces of soy cheese on the bread to make a sandwich. Place the sandwich in the skillet. Both sides of the sandwich should be golden brown, and the cheese melted. If the bread is starting to brown too quickly, lower the heat to give the soy cheese a chance to melt.

Rock 'n' Roll Reuben

Makes 1 sandwich

RUSSIAN DRESSING

½ cup Nayonnaise

¼ cup sugar-free ketchup

1 tablespoon white wine vinegar

1 tablespoon minced onion

Dash of dry mustard

Salt and pepper or Spike

2 slices rye bread

2 to 3 ounces soy Swiss cheese

2 to 3 ounces soy pastrami

¼ cup organic sauerkraut

1 tablespoon soy margarine

In a small bowl, mix all the ingredients for the dressing and set aside.

Make a sandwich out of the bread, Russian dressing, soy cheese, soy pastrami, and sauerkraut. Melt the soy margarine in a small skillet over medium heat. Place the sandwich in the skillet and cover it with a heavy lid. Cook until golden brown. Flip and cook the other side until the soy cheese is melted.

Rachel's Rockin' Turkey Roll-up

Serves 1

1 to 2 tablespoons Nayonnaise

1 large whole wheat tortilla

4 thin slices free-range turkey

¼ organic avocado, thinly sliced

2 slices organic tomato

1 to 2 large organic lettuce leaves

Spread the Nayonnaise on the tortilla. Layer the turkey, avocado, tomato, and lettuce. Roll up and eat.

Mary Beth's
Antipasto Sandwich

Serves 6

1 large baguette or 1 loaf Italian bread

1 jar (4 ounces) black olive paste

2 small jars (16 to 24 ounces) artichoke
   hearts, chopped

1 jar (8 ounces) roasted red peppers,
   or 2 large red peppers, roasted,
   sliced in strips

1 bunch arugula, washed and spun dry

Slice the bread in half horizontally. Scoop out some of the bread from the top and bottom. Spread the top and bottom with the black olive paste. Layer the artichoke hearts, pepper strips, and arugula over the bottom. Replace the top, wrap in foil, and refrigerate about 4 hours. Slice on the diagonal and serve.

Burgers

Serves 4

1 pound free-range ground turkey
    or ground soy meat
2 tablespoons Spike
1 tablespoon olive oil
4 slices soy cheese
Whole grain burger buns

Mix the turkey or soy meat with Spike. With your hands, form the ground beef or ground soy into 4 patties. Heat a nonstick frying pan on high heat. Drizzle a little olive oil in the pan. Put the patties in and fry until browned on one side, about 2 to 3 minutes. Turn the patties over and cook for another 2 to 3 minutes. Turn off the heat and top with soy cheese. Tuck the patties into buns and serve.

VARIATIONS

Create your own burger. Add soy bacon, vegetarian chili, ketchup, Nayonnaise, mustard, relish, organic tomato slices, sliced onion, pickles, or organic lettuce.

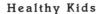

Dylan Digs Pizza

Makes 2 pizzas

THE SAUCE

1½ tablespoons olive oil

1 small organic onion, chopped

1 clove garlic, minced

1 can (15 ounces) organic tomato puree

¼ cup water

1½ teaspoons Sucanat

1 teaspoon dried oregano

1½ teaspoons dried basil

Dash of Spike

Make the sauce: Heat the oil in a large saucepan over medium heat. Add the onions and cook until translucent, about 3 minutes. Add the garlic and sauté 1 more minute, stirring constantly. Add the tomato puree, water, Sucanat, oregano, basil, and Spike. Bring the mixture to a boil, lower the heat, and simmer, stirring occasionally, for 30 minutes. While the sauce is simmering, make the dough.

1 package (¼ ounce) active dry yeast

1 teaspoon Sucanat or honey

1 cup warm water

2 tablespoons olive oil

1 teaspoon salt

2½ cups unbleached whole wheat flour

8 ounces soy mozzarella cheese

Olive oil for greasing

Cornmeal for sprinkling

Whole wheat flour

¼ cup soy Parmesan

Put the yeast and Sucanat in a large bowl. Add warm water and stir until the yeast dissolves. Stir in the oil, salt, and flour. When the dough becomes stiff, flour your hands and a work surface. Knead the dough for 8 to 10 minutes, adding flour to keep it from sticking, until smooth and elastic. Dust the dough with flour and put it on a plate. Cover with a towel and let rise for 1 to 2 hours, until it doubles in size. Use the dough within 30 minutes.

Preheat the oven to 500 degrees. Shred the soy mozzarella. Grease 2 pizza pans with oil. Sprinkle the pans with cornmeal. Dust your hands with flour and divide the dough in half. With your hands, form each half into a ball. Put on a pizza pan and press into a round. With your fingers, pinch a little ridge on the edge of dough. Do the same with the other ball of dough. Spread half of the sauce on each pizza dough. Because soy cheese tends to cook quickly, bake the dough with the sauce for 5 minutes prior to adding the cheese. Sprinkle the pizzas with the cheese and bake for 1 minute, making sure it's melted and the crust is golden brown.

Quesadillas with an Attitude

Makes 8 to 16 servings

4 tablespoons cooking oil

Eight 8-inch whole wheat tortillas

1 cup grated soy cheddar cheese

8 slices organic tomato (optional)

1 organic avocado, sliced (optional)

1 tablespoon soy sour cream (optional)

Heat 1 tablespoon oil in a medium skillet over medium heat for 1 minute. Place a tortilla in the skillet. Top with ¼ cup soy cheese and a couple of slices each of the tomato and avocado, if using. Cover with another tortilla. Cook about 2 minutes, until the soy cheese begins to melt. Flip and cook another 2 to 3 minutes. Repeat three times with remaining tortillas. Cut into wedges and garnish with soy sour cream, if using.

Enchiladas

Serves 4 to 6

1 pound free-range ground turkey or
   ground soy meat
Cooking oil, as needed
1 medium organic onion, chopped
1 cup soy sour cream
2 cups soy cheddar cheese, shredded
2 tablespoons chopped fresh parsley
¼ teaspoon pepper
½ cup water
1 tablespoon chili powder
½ teaspoon dried oregano
¼ teaspoon ground cumin
1 clove garlic, minced
1 can organic tomato sauce
8 corn tortillas

Preheat the oven to 350 degrees. In a large skillet over medium heat, brown the meat, stirring occasionally, for about 8 to 10 minutes. If using soy meat, you may need to oil the pan a little first so it doesn't stick. Drain. Stir in the onion, ½ cup soy sour cream, 1 cup soy cheese, parsley, and pepper. Cover and set aside. In a small saucepan, combine the water, chili powder, oregano, cumin, garlic, and tomato sauce over medium heat until it simmers, stirring occasionally. Reduce the heat and simmer for 5 minutes. Pour into an ungreased pie dish.

Dip each tortilla into the sauce, coating both sides. Spoon about ¼ cup turkey or soy meat mixture into each tortilla. Roll the tortillas around the filling. Put in an ungreased rectangular baking dish. Pour the remaining sauce over enchiladas. Bake, uncovered, for 20 minutes. Remove. Sprinkle the remaining soy cheese over the top and garnish with the remaining soy sour cream.

Taylor's Taco Salad

Serves 4

1 head organic romaine lettuce
2 organic tomatoes
1 medium red onion
1 pound free-range ground turkey or
   ground soy meat
1 tablespoon canola oil
½ cup bottled all-natural chili sauce
½ cup vegetable stock or water
1 teaspoon chili powder
¾ teaspoon salt or Spike
½ teaspoon ground cumin
2 tablespoons all-natural Italian
   salad dressing
1 cup soy cheddar cheese
All-natural tortilla chips

Chop the lettuce into bite-sized pieces. Chop the tomatoes into bite-sized pieces. Cut the onion into quarters. Thinly slice 1 quarter and add to a salad bowl with the lettuce and tomato. Chop the remaining onion and set aside.

In a large skillet, sauté the meat in the oil until it loses its red color, about 5 minutes. Add the chili sauce, stock, chili powder, salt, and cumin. Stir well. Reduce the heat to medium and cook about 10 minutes, stirring often.

Add the Italian dressing to the salad and toss with a large spoon. Spoon the meat mixture on top of the salad. Sprinkle with cheese and remaining onions. Surround the bowl with tortilla chips and serve.

Fabulous Fajitas

Serves 4

Juice of 2 large organic limes
⅓ cup olive oil
½ teaspoon dried oregano
½ teaspoon ground cumin
½ teaspoon Spike
¼ teaspoon chili powder
4 boneless, skinless, free-range chicken breasts
   or soy chicken breasts
4 large whole wheat flour tortillas

To a small mixing bowl, add the lime juice, olive oil, oregano, cumin, Spike, and chili powder. Mix the ingredients until blended. Put the chicken in a large bowl. Pour the mixture over the chicken and turn until all sides are coated. Cover with plastic wrap and marinate in the refrigerator for at least 1 hour. When ready to cook, preheat the broiler on high.

Remove the chicken from the bowl and broil until chicken is browned, about 5 to 7 minutes. Flip and cook another 5 to 7 minutes. Preheat the oven to 400 degrees, or if the oven and broiler are the same, let the oven cool to 400 degrees. Wrap the tortillas in foil and place in the oven for 5 to 10 minutes.

Cut the chicken into strips and put in a bowl. Place some of the chicken, guacamole, salsa, and soy sour cream on each tortilla. Wrap and serve.

Kooky Chili Billy con Carne

Serves 6

1 medium onion, chopped

2 tablespoons olive oil

1½ pounds free-range ground turkey or
ground soy meat

1 can (16 ounces) crushed organic tomatoes

1 can (16 ounces) kidney beans, drained

1 can organic tomato sauce

2 teaspoons chili powder

1 teaspoon Spike

1 teaspoon Sucanat or agave extract

½ teaspoon ground cumin

GARNISHES

Grated soy cheese

Chopped onion

Tortilla chips

To a skillet over medium-high heat, add the onion and olive oil and sauté about 3 minutes. Add the turkey or soy meat. Cook, while breaking it up, until it loses all the pink color. Lower the heat to medium-low and add the tomatoes in their juices, kidney beans, tomato sauce, chili powder, Spike, Sucanat, and cumin, stirring well. Cover and simmer, stirring occasionally, for about 1 hour. Serve in a bowl with some grated soy cheese or onion and tortilla chips.

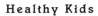

Not So Chilly Chile Lentil

Serves 10

3½ cups water

3 cups vegetable stock

2½ cups dried lentils

1½ tablespoons olive oil

2½ cups chopped organic celery

3 tablespoons tamari sauce

2 tablespoons chili powder

1½ tablespoons ground cumin

2 teaspoons dried basil

1 can (8 ounces) Spanish-style organic
   tomato sauce

1 can (7 ounces) mild green chiles

1 can (28 ounces) whole peeled organic
   tomatoes, chopped, and their juices

2 teaspoons Spike

Salt to taste

In a 5- or 6-quart pot, bring to a boil the water, vegetable stock, lentils, olive oil, and celery. Cover and simmer 35 minutes. Add the tamari, chili powder, cumin, and basil. Continue simmering until the lentils are soft, about 20 minutes. Stir occasionally.

In a blender, blend the tomato sauce with the chiles until smooth. Add to the soup, along with the tomatoes and their juice. Add the Spike and salt to taste. Simmer 15 minutes, stirring occasionally. The consistency should be medium-thick. Add water if needed, and serve.

Mary Beth's Really Yummy Pasta

Serves 4

I'm telling you, I have never felt such love as I did when I served this dish. I am trying to decide who to have over so I can hear the accolades all over again.

—MARY BETH

2 tablespoons olive oil

5 large cloves garlic, coarsely chopped

1 can (28 ounces) whole peeled tomatoes,
   coarsely chopped, juice reserved

1 can (15 ounces) tomato sauce,
   such as Muir Glen

2 jars brine-cured black olives,
   drained, pitted, and sliced

1 pound fettuccine

1 tablespoon Sucanat (optional)

1 bunch fresh basil, washed and torn

Heat the olive oil in a skillet over medium heat. Sauté the garlic, being careful not to let it brown. Add the chopped tomatoes and sauté for a few minutes. Add the juice from the tomatoes and the tomato sauce. Toss in the olives and simmer the mixture for minutes.

Boil water in a large pot and cook the pasta. You might wish to add a little Sucanat to the sauce at this point to cut the acidity. During the last 5 minutes of cooking time, add the basil. Drain. Pour the sauce over the pasta.

Pasta Primavera

Makes 4 servings

1½ cups vegetable stock
2 sprigs fresh thyme
Pinch of salt
½ cup peeled and diced organic carrots
½ cup organic cauliflower florets
1 cup organic broccoli florets
½ cup organic peas
1 pound penne pasta
2 tablespoons olive oil
1 cup soy Parmesan cheese

Bring a large pot of water to a boil.

In a medium skillet, bring 1 cup of the stock to a boil. Add the thyme and salt. Add the carrots, cauliflower, and broccoli. Cook about 6 to 7 minutes. Add the peas and cook until all the veggies are tender, about 2 or 3 more minutes. Turn off the heat.

Salt the boiling water and cook the pasta according to the directions on the package. When the pasta is just about done, reheat the vegetables over medium heat, stirring in the olive oil. Cook about 1 minute. Add the remaining ½ cup stock. Drain the pasta and toss with the vegetables. Top with the soy Parmesan and serve.

Creamy Fettuccine

Makes 4 servings

10 ounces fresh organic spinach,
   trimmed, rinsed, and drained
4 tablespoons soy margarine
Salt and pepper
1 cup soy cream
1 pound fettuccine
1 cup soy Parmesan cheese

Bring a large pot of water to a boil. Chop the spinach coarsely. Over medium heat, melt 2 tablespoons margarine in a large skillet with a lid. Add the spinach, salt, and pepper. Cover, lower the heat, and cook, stirring occasionally, until the spinach is tender, about 10 minutes. Uncover and add ½ cup soy cream. Cook approximately 5 minutes more.

Salt the boiling water and cook the pasta according to the directions on the package. When it is just about done, put the remaining 2 tablespoons margarine in a large warm bowl and add 2 tablespoons cooking water. Drain the pasta and toss with the margarine and ½ cup soy Parmesan in the large bowl. Add the spinach sauce and serve. Put the remaining soy Parmesan on the table for passing.

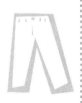

Turkey Bolognese

Serves 10

2 teaspoons olive oil

1 medium organic white onion,
   chopped

4 cloves garlic, chopped

1 tablespoon dried marjoram

3 teaspoons dried basil

2 teaspoons fennel seeds

1 pound free-range ground turkey

2 cans (28 ounces each) crushed
   organic tomatoes

½ cup white wine or vegetable stock

1 box penne or spaghetti

Soy Parmesan for garnishing

Add the oil to a large skillet over medium heat. When hot, add the onion, garlic, and herbs. Cook until the onions are golden, about 3 to 5 minutes, stirring occasionally. Add the turkey and cook until it loses its raw color. Add the tomatoes and wine, and cook, uncovered, over low heat, stirring occasionally, about 2 to 2½ hours. Bring a large pot of water to a boil and cook the pasta according to the directions on the package. Toss with the sauce, garnish with soy Parmesan, and serve.

Sydney's Saucy Spaghetti and "Meatballs"

Serves 4

12 ounces to 1 pound free-range ground turkey or Gimme Lean (sausage flavor)

1 cage-free egg

1 cup soy Parmesan

½ cup chopped fresh parsley

1 teaspoon minced garlic

½ cup fresh breadcrumbs or wheat germ

Salt to taste

Olive oil

SYDNEY'S SAUCE

1 tablespoon olive oil

3 shallots, chopped

4 cloves garlic, chopped

1 can (35 ounces) whole organic plum tomatoes, drained and pulp squeezed dry

1 tablespoon dried basil

1 can (28 ounces) crushed organic tomatoes

½ cup vegetable stock

Spaghetti

In a medium bowl, lightly mix the "meat," egg, half of the Parmesan, the parsley, garlic, breadcrumbs, and salt. Form into balls.

Heat the olive oil for about 3 minutes in a large skillet over medium heat. Add the meatballs and cook, continually turning so they don't stick to the skillet, for about 15 minutes, or until they are browned. Remove from the pan and set aside. (You can also buy premade turkey balls and soy meatballs.)

Make the sauce: Add the oil to a large skillet over medium heat. When the oil is hot, add the shallots and garlic. Cook for 1 or 2 minutes, making sure the garlic doesn't burn. Add the plum tomatoes and mash. Add the basil, crushed tomatoes, and stock. Simmer about 5 minutes. Add the "meat" balls. Cook for 1 to 2 minutes. Put on top of cooked spaghetti, prepared according to the directions on the package. Pass the remaining ½ cup Parmesan at the table.

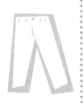

Lasagna

Serves 8

1 pound ground turkey or ground soy meat
  (sausage flavor)
1 small organic onion, diced
Olive oil, as needed
1 can (28 ounces) organic tomatoes and their juices
1 can (12 ounces) organic tomato paste
2 teaspoons maple sugar
½ teaspoon dried oregano
½ teaspoon dried thyme
¼ teaspoon garlic powder
Salt or Spike
1 bay leaf
1 pound lasagna noodles
2 pounds firm tofu, crumbled with a fork
2 cage-free eggs
1 pound soy mozzarella, diced

In a large pot over high heat, cook the ground turkey or soy meat and onion until the meat is browned. (If using soy meat, you may need a little olive oil.) Add the tomatoes, tomato paste, maple sugar, oregano, thyme, garlic powder, salt, and bay leaf. Heat until boiling, stirring to break up the tomatoes. Reduce the heat to low and simmer, stirring occasionally, about 30 minutes. Discard the bay leaf. Remove any excess fat from the top of the sauce.

Preheat the oven to 375 degrees. In a large pot of boiling water, cook the lasagna noodles according to the directions on the package. Drain well. In a 13-by-9-inch baking dish, arrange half of the drained noodles, overlapping them to fit in the dish. In a medium bowl, combine the tofu and eggs. Spoon half over the noodles. Sprinkle with half of the soy cheese, and top with half of the sauce. Repeat the layers. Bake for 45 minutes. Cool 10 minutes before serving.

Rockin' Rice and Rye

Serves 6

2 cups brown rice
1 cup rye berries
3 cups water
3 cups vegetable broth
2 small organic carrots, chopped
1 organic celery stalk, chopped
½ organic onion, chopped
1½ cups frozen organic green beans
½ cup water
Bragg Liquid Aminos

In a large saucepan, mix the brown rice, rye, water, vegetable broth, carrots, celery, and onion. Bring to a boil. Lower the heat and simmer 20 to 25 minutes, until the rice and rye are tender and have absorbed the liquid.

In a small saucepan, bring the green beans and water to a boil. Cook for 2 minutes and drain. Combine rice and rye with the green beans and season with Bragg Liquid Aminos.

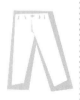

Couscous with Raisins

Makes 4 servings

2¼ cups plus ⅓ cup vegetable stock
1 cinnamon stick
½ teaspoon minced fresh ginger
Salt and pepper to taste
⅓ cup raisins
4 tablespoons soy margarine
½ cup pine nuts
1½ cups couscous
Minced fresh parsley (optional)

In a small pan, warm 2¼ cups of the vegetable stock with the cinnamon, ginger, salt, and pepper over low heat. Heat the remaining ⅓ cup stock and soak the raisins.

Melt 1 tablespoon margarine in a small skillet over medium heat. Add the pine nuts and cook, stirring occasionally, until light brown, about 5 minutes. Set aside. In a medium pan over medium-low heat, melt 2 tablespoons soy margarine. Add the couscous and cook about 1 minute. Strain the stock and add it to the couscous. Bring it to a boil and reduce the heat to low. Cover and cook until all the liquid is absorbed, about 5 to 8 minutes.

Drain the raisins and gently add them to the couscous mixture, along with the pine nuts and remaining 1 tablespoon soy margarine. Add the fresh parsley, if desired. Fluff with a fork and serve.

Sautéed Scallops on Rice

Serves 3 to 4

3 tablespoons soy margarine

3 scallions, chopped

1 large clove garlic, pressed

Grated fresh ginger

1 medium organic zucchini,
  chopped

1 organic celery stalk,
  chopped

1 pound scallops

½ cup pine nuts

Salt and pepper to taste

3 tablespoons light soy sauce

2 tablespoons Dijon
  mustard

2 cups cooked brown rice

In a large skillet melt the margarine over medium heat and sauté the vegetables for 5 minutes. Add the scallops and all the other ingredients except the rice. Sauté 10 minutes. Serve over the brown rice.

Flounder

Serves 4

2 pounds flounder

1 organic lemon

1 cup soy sour cream

1 teaspoon minced fresh dill

2 scallions, chopped

Preheat the oven to 450 degrees. Wash the fish, pat dry, and put in a baking pan. Squeeze the lemon over it. In a small bowl, mix the soy sour cream, dill, and scallions. Spread evenly over the fish. Bake for 10 minutes, then place under the broiler for 5 minutes. Serve.

Whitefish

Serves 3 to 4

Soy margarine
1½ pounds whitefish fillets
1 organic lemon
2 tablespoons light tamari sauce
½ cup breadcrumbs
1 teaspoon Spike

Preheat the oven to 350 degrees. Grease a baking dish with soy margarine. Wash and dry the fish. Put on a large plate. Squeeze the lemon over it and sprinkle with tamari. Put breadcrumbs and Spike in a large plastic bag. Put the fillets in the bag, one at a time, and shake to coat evenly.

Place the fish in the baking dish and put a little dab of soy margarine on top. Bake until flaky, about 30 minutes.

Fish Florentine

Serves 4

Soy margarine
2 pounds mild-flavored fish fillets, such as
    flounder, whitefish, or sole
1 pound fresh organic spinach,
    washed and drained
1 cup soy sour cream
½ cup chopped scallions
1 organic lemon, halved
½ cup wheat germ or breadcrumbs
1 teaspoon sesame seeds
½ cup grated soy cheddar cheese

Preheat the oven to 350 degrees. Grease a casserole dish with soy margarine. Lay half of the fish on the bottom of the casserole dish. Squeeze a lemon half over the fish. Lightly cook the spinach and drain it.

In a medium bowl, mix the spinach, soy sour cream, and scallions. Spread this mixture over the fish in the casserole. Place the remaining fish over the spinach mixture. Squeeze the remaining lemon half over the top of the fish. Sprinkle with wheat germ, sesame seeds, and soy cheese. Bake for 30 minutes and serve.

Barbecued Chicken

Serves 6

¼ cup soy margarine
One 2- to 3-pound free-range
   organic chicken
1 tablespoon olive oil
1 medium organic onion, chopped
2 cloves garlic, minced
½ cup rice vinegar
1½ cups organic ketchup
1 tablespoon Dijon mustard
2 tablespoon maple sugar
¼ cup fresh organic lemon juice

Preheat the oven to 375 degrees. Heat the soy margarine in a 13-by-9-by-2-inch rectangular pan. Place chicken in the margarine, turning to coat. Place, breast side down in the pan. Bake, uncovered, for 30 minutes.

Heat the oil in a medium saucepan over medium heat. Add the onion and garlic and cook for about 5 minutes, stirring occasionally. Add the remaining ingredients, lower the heat, and simmer for 5 to 10 minutes. Remove from the heat.

Drain the fat from the chicken. Turn it breast side up and spoon the sauce over the chicken. Bake, uncovered, until the thickest pieces are tender and the juices of the chicken run clear, about 30 minutes.

Lemon Chicken

Serves 4

½ cup soy margarine
¼ cup fresh organic lemon
  juice
1 teaspoon Spike

1 teaspoon raw cane sugar
¼ teaspoon pepper
2½- to 3-pound free-range
  organic chicken, quartered

Preheat the broiler. To a medium saucepan, add all the ingredients except the chicken. Heat until the margarine is melted. Place the chicken skin side down in a large broiling pan. Baste with margarine mixture. Broil the chicken 20 minutes, basting with the margarine mixture. Turn the chicken and broil another 15 to 20 minutes. Check for doneness frequently by pricking the largest breast at the fattest point: The meat should be fully opaque with no traces of red. Remove and serve.

Nicky and Joey's Famous Fried Chicken

Makes 4 to 6 servings

½ cup olive or vegetable oil
2 cups unbleached flour
1 tablespoon kosher salt
1 teaspoon black pepper
2 tablespoons ground cinnamon
3 to 4 pounds free-range chicken, cut up and excess fat trimmed

Add the olive oil to a deep skillet over medium-high heat. Mix the flour and seasonings in a paper bag. Toss the chicken, 2 to 3 pieces at a time, in the bag until well coated. Set aside on cooking rack.

When the oil reaches 350 degrees, add the chicken skin side down and cover. Cook for about 7 minutes. Uncover, turn, and cook for another 7 minutes. Turn again and cook for 5 minutes. Drain on paper towels to absorb the excess oil and serve.

Chicken Fingers

Makes 4 servings

1½ pounds boneless, skinless free-range
    chicken breast or tenders,
    rinsed and patted dry
1½ cups plain soy yogurt
1 cup olive oil
Unbleached flour for coating
Salt and pepper or Spike

Cut the chicken into 2-inch strips. Marinate them in the soy yogurt until ready to use.

Heat the oil in a skillet over medium-high heat. In a shallow dish, season the flour with salt and pepper. When the oil in the skillet reaches 350 degrees, raise the heat to high. Coat the chicken pieces in the flour mixture and place them in the oil. Cook about 2 to 3 minutes per side, until brown. Drain on paper towels and serve.

DESSERTS

Apple à la Mode

Serves 2

1 organic apple, unpeeled, cored and cut into quarters
1 tablespoon soy margarine
¼ cup raw organic sugar
1 tablespoon cinnamon
¼ cup granola
1 scoop soy ice cream or Rice Dream

In a microwave-safe bowl, place the apple skin side down. Pat a little of the margarine on each quarter. Sprinkle the tops with sugar, cinnamon, and granola. Microwave on high until the apple is soft, about 1 minute. Top with a dollop of soy ice cream.

Pudding Please!

Serves 4

⅓ cup Sucanat or maple sugar
1½ tablespoons arrowroot
1 cup grain-sweetened chocolate chips or carob chips
2 cups soy milk
1 teaspoon vanilla extract

In a medium saucepan, combine the Sucanat and arrowroot. Turn the heat to medium. Add the chips and milk, and cook, stirring constantly, until the pudding is thick, about 6 minutes. Remove from the heat. Stir in the vanilla and let cool, stirring occasionally. Spoon into 4 serving dishes and refrigerate for about 1 hour.

Checkerboard Birthday Cake

Makes 1 cake

¾ cup soy margarine at room temperature, plus extra
   for greasing
2¼ cups unbleached flour
2 teaspoons baking powder
½ teaspoon salt
¾ cup plus 1 tablespoon soy milk
1½ teaspoons vanilla extract
1½ cups unprocessed pure cane sugar
3 large cage-free eggs
¼ cup grain-sweetened chocolate chips, melted
⅛ cup unsweetened chocolate, melted
Chocolate Frosting (recipe follows)

Preheat the oven to 350 degrees. Grease three 8-inch round cake pans. Line the bottoms with wax paper, grease the paper, and dust the pans with flour.

In a medium bowl, mix the flour, baking powder, and salt. Put the ¾ cup soy milk and vanilla in a small bowl. In the bowl of an electric mixer, cream the ¾ cup soy margarine and the sugar for at least 5 minutes, until nice and creamy. Lower the speed to medium-low and add the eggs, one at a time. Reduce the speed to low. Add the flour mixture alternately with the milk mixture. Beat until smooth.

Spoon half of the batter neatly into a Ziploc bag, trying to keep the batter to one side of the bag at the bottom, as if you were filling a pastry bag. Add the melted chocolate and remaining 1 tablespoon of soy milk to the remaining batter. Spoon into another Ziploc bag. Cut off 1 inch from the corner of each bag to create an opening. Pipe a 1½-inch-wide band of chocolate batter around 2 cake pans. Squeeze a 1½-inch-wide band of vanilla next to each chocolate band. Add enough chocolate to fill in the center of the two pans so that the whole cake pan is full. In the third pan, repeat the rings, but start and end with vanilla. When assembled, the cake will have a checkerboard look.

Stagger the cake pans in the oven on two racks. Bake for 20 minutes. Test the cakes with a toothpick. It should come out almost clean. Cool on wire racks for

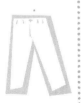

about 10 minutes. With a thin knife, loosen the layers and invert them onto a wire rack. Remove the wax paper and cool.

Place one layer with the chocolate on the outside on a cake plate. Spread with ½ cup of the frosting. Place the layer with the vanilla on the outside on top and frost. Top with the third layer and finish frosting the cake.

CHOCOLATE FROSTING
¾ cup Sucanat
¼ cup unbleached white flour
3 tablespoons unsweetened cocoa
1 cup soy cream
1 cup soy margarine at room temperature
1 tablespoon vanilla extract
½ cup grain-sweetened chocolate, melted and cooled

In a medium saucepan, stir together the Sucanat, flour, and cocoa until well blended. Slowly stir in the soy cream and continue stirring until smooth. Cook over medium heat, stirring, until the mixture thickens and boils. Reduce the heat to low. Cook 2 minutes, stirring constantly. Remove from heat and cool completely. In the bowl of an electric mixer, beat the margarine at medium speed until creamy. Slowly add the cooled soy cream mixture. Add the vanilla and melted chocolate and blend well. You may have to refrigerate the frosting a little for a stiffer, more spreadable consistency.

Carrot Cake

Makes 1 cake

2½ cups unbleached flour

1 teaspoon baking powder

2 teaspoons baking soda

2 teaspoons cinnamon

1 teaspoon salt

½ teaspoon ground nutmeg

4 large cage-free eggs

1 cup Sucanat

¾ cup maple sugar

¼ cup soy milk

1 tablespoon vanilla extract

1 cup canola oil

3 cups lightly packed
shredded organic carrots

1 cup chopped walnuts
(optional)

FROSTING

2 tubs (8 ounces each) soy cream cheese

½ cup honey

1 teaspoon vanilla extract

Preheat the oven to 350 degrees. Grease a 13-by-11-inch metal baking pan. Line the bottom with wax paper. Grease the paper and dust with flour.

In a medium bowl, mix the flour, baking powder, baking soda, cinnamon, salt, and nutmeg and set aside. In the bowl of an electric mixer, beat the eggs and sugars at medium speed for about 2 minutes. Beat in the soy milk and vanilla.

Reduce the speed to low, add the flour mixture, and beat until smooth. Fold in the carrots and walnuts, if desired, by hand. (Kids might like it more without the nuts.) Pour the batter into the pan. Bake 55 to 60 minutes. Cool on a wire rack for 10 minutes. With a small knife loosen the cake from the sides of the pan; invert onto a rack and let cool.

Remove wax paper. Make the frosting while the cake is baking: Cream together the ingredients and refrigerate for a short time to stiffen. Frost the cake when cooled.

Brownies

Makes 1 dozen

¾ cup soy margarine, plus extra for greasing the pan

½ cup unsweetened dairy-free chocolate chips

½ cup grain-sweetened chocolate chips

2 cups Sucanat

1 tablespoon vanilla extract

5 large cage-free eggs, beaten

1½ cups unbleached white flour

½ teaspoon salt

Preheat the oven to 350 degrees. Grease a 13-by-9-inch metal baking pan. In a large saucepan, melt the soy margarine and all the chocolate chips over low heat, stirring frequently. Remove from the heat. Stir in the Sucanat and vanilla. Beat in the eggs and blend well.

In a small bowl, combine the flour and salt. Stir into the chocolate mixture until just blended. Pour into the baking pan and spread evenly. Bake for 30 minutes. Cool in the pan. When cool, cut and remove.

Blondies

Makes 2 dozen

6 tablespoons soy margarine, plus extra
   for greasing the pan
¾ cup maple sugar
1 cup Sucanat
2 teaspoons vanilla extract
2 large cage-free eggs
1 cup unbleached flour
2 teaspoons baking powder
1 teaspoon salt
1½ cups coarsely chopped pecans

Preheat the oven to 350 degrees. Grease a 13-by-9-inch metal baking pan. In a large saucepan, melt the margarine over low heat. Stir in the maple sugar, Sucanat, and vanilla. Beat in the eggs. In a small bowl, mix the flour, baking powder, and salt. Combine the wet and dry ingredients and stir in the pecans.

   Pour the batter into the pan and spread out evenly. Bake for 30 minutes. Cool completely in the pan on a wire rack. When cool, cut and remove.

Peanut Butter Cookies

Makes 4 dozen

½ cup soy margarine, plus extra for greasing the cookie sheets

1½ cups unbleached flour

½ teaspoon baking soda

½ cup creamy or crunchy all-natural peanut butter

½ cup Sucanat

½ cup maple sugar

1 large cage-free egg

½ teaspoon vanilla extract

Preheat the oven to 375 degrees. Grease 2 large cookie sheets. In a small bowl, combine the flour and baking soda. In the bowl of an electric mixer on low speed, beat the soy margarine until creamy. Add the peanut butter, Sucanat, and maple sugar. Beat until well blended. Beat in the egg and vanilla. Reduce the speed to low and add half of the flour mixture. Beat until well blended and add the rest of the flour mixture. Mix with a wooden spoon.

Form the dough into 1-inch balls and place 2 inches apart on the cookie sheets. Use a fork to press the cookies down. Bake for 10 minutes and cool.

Oatmeal Cookies

Makes 4 dozen

8 ounces soy margarine at room temperature

¾ cup Sucanat

¾ cup maple sugar

2 large cage-free eggs at room temperature

1 tablespoon vanilla extract

1 tablespoon water

1¾ cups unbleached flour

1 teaspoon baking soda

½ teaspoon salt

2½ cups rolled oats

1 cup shredded coconut

Preheat the oven to 375 degrees. Cream the margarine, Sucanat, and maple sugar in a large bowl. Add the eggs, vanilla, and water, and mix thoroughly. In another bowl, mix the flour, baking soda, salt, oats, and coconut. Combine the ingredients. Put heaping tablespoons of dough on a cookie sheet and bake 12 minutes.

Chocolate Chip Cookies

Makes 4 dozen cookies

8 ounces soy margarine at room temperature,
  plus extra for greasing cookie sheet

¾ cup maple sugar

1 cup Sucanat

2 large cage-free eggs

1 teaspoon vanilla extract

2 cups unbleached flour

¾ teaspoon baking soda

1 teaspoon salt

2 cups grain-sweetened chocolate chips

Preheat the oven to 350 degrees. Lightly grease the cookie sheet. Cream the soy margarine and sugars in a large bowl until light. Add the eggs and vanilla. Do not overbeat. Stir in the dry ingredients and mix well. Stir in the chips. Drop large tablespoons of dough onto the cookie sheet. Bake 12 minutes.

············

Appendix

Marilu's Shopping List for Healthy Kids

Snacks

Nuts

Raisins, dried cranberries (no sulfites)

Kettle Chips: Mesquite, Sea Salt & Vinegar, Honey Dijon, Regular, Lightly Salted

Garden of Eatin Potato Chips

Garden of Eatin Tortilla Chips: Chili & Lime, Blue Corn, Salsa, Yellow Corn, Black Bean

Newman's Own Organic Pretzels

Hain Food Group, Inc., Rice Cakes: Honey Nut, Popcorn, Peanut Butter

Trader Joe's Organic Tortilla Chips: Blue Corn, Yellow Corn, Black Bean

Trader Joe's "Hawaiian Justice" Potato Chips: Honey Mustard, Salt Free, Habeas Crispus

Trader Joe's Pretzels

Trader Joe's Rice Cakes

Santa Cruz Organic Applesauce

Whole Foods Applesauce

Whole Soy Yogurt

Breakfast Foods

Barbara's Breakfast Cereals: Shredded Spoonfuls, Puffins (Regular & Cinnamon)

Van's Brand Waffles: Belgian, Regular, Blueberry

Trader Joe's Wheat Free Toaster Waffles

Amy's Toaster Treats: Apple, Strawberry

Quick Meals

Health and Wealth Veggie Munchies Toaster Treats: Spinach Tofu, Pizza Tofu, Veggie Munchies, Pizza Munchies, Supreme, Spinach

Hain Food Group, Inc., Pizsoy

Health & Wealth Chicken Nuggets

Natural Food Systems Natural Sea Fish Sticks, Fish Patties

Amy's Soy Pizza

Amy's Vegetable Soy Cheese Pizza

Amy's Macaroni & Cheese

Amy's Veggie Loaf

Cascadian Farms Vegetables & Fries

Grandma Mallina's Organic Spagettios

Imagine Soups

Boca Burgers

Yves Tofu & Veggie Dogs

Shelton's Chicken Franks

Whole Foods Turkey and Chicken Dogs

Organic Food Products, Inc., Organic Kid's Meals

Beverages/Milk Substitutes

White Wave-Silk

Silk Soy Milk

Soy ½ & ½

Imagine Foods: Rice Dream Rice Milk: Original Enriched, Vanilla Enriched, Chocolate Enriched, Carob Enriched, Original, Vanilla, Chocolate, Carob

"Soy-Dream" Soy Milk: Assorted Flavors

"Power-Dream" Meal Shakes: Assorted Flavors

Trader Joe's "Soy Um" Soy Milk

Trader Joe's "Rice Um" Rice Milk

Knudsen Spritzers

Knudsen Juices

Cheese Substitutes

Soyco Foods "Light n' Less" Soy Veggy Singles: Mozzarella, Swiss, American, Jalapeño Jack, Provolone

Sweet Treats

Candy

    Panda Licorice: Raspberry, Strawberry, Traditional Black Licorice

    Tropical Source Chocolate Bars

Cookies/Doughnuts

    Uncle Eddie's Vegan Cookies: Trail Mix, Oatmeal, Chocolate Chip Peanut Butter, Chocolate Chip

    "No" Cookies: Oatmeal, Peanut Butter, Chocolate Chip

Hain Food Group, Inc., Graham Crackers: Plain, Cinnamon
Health Valley Animal or Graham Crackers
Frookie's Sandwich Cookies: Chocolate, Vanilla, Chocolate & Vanilla Sandwich, Peanut Butter, Lemon
Donut & Cookie Bakery, Inc., Eggless Donut: Plain, Carob Covered, Vanilla, Chocolate/Chocolate
Ice Cream/Puddings/Popsicles:
Tofutti Cuties: Chocolate, Vanilla, Peanut Butter
Soy Delicious: Chocolate, Vanilla, Peanut Butter/Chocolate (Marilu recommends)
Rice Dream Ice Cream
Whole Soy Ice Cream Sandwiches & Ice Cream Bars
Imagine Puddings: Butterscotch, Banana, Chocolate, Lemon
Sweet Nothings Frozen Desserts
Fruitfull Popsicles

Snacks
Robert's American Gourmet: Veggie Booty, Fruity Booty, Spirulina Spirals, Power Puffs, Smart Puffs
Guiltless Gourmet: Baked chips, Fat-free Bean Dips
Kettle Chips: Sea Salt & Vinegar, Honey Dijon, Salsa, Salt and Ground Pepper, Krinkle Cut, Lightly Salted
Good Health: Veggie Sticks
Newman's Own: Popcorn
Whole Foods Bread Spread: Olive, Artichoke

Breakfast Foods
New Morning: Fruit-e-O's
Mother's: Groovy Grahams, Honey Round-Ups, Peanut Butter Bumpers, Cinnamon Oat Crunch
Kashi: Chocolate Pillows, Honey Puffed, Medley
U.S. Mills: Cocomotion
Barbara's: Honey Crunch Stars, Cocoa Crunch, Brown rice crisps
Erewhon Oatmeal: Maple Spice, Apple Cinnamon

Quick Meals
Fantastic Soups
Amy's organic soups: No Chicken Noodle, Lentil, Vegetable
Tasty Bite: Bengal Lentils, Jodhpur Lentils, Simla Potatoes

Beverages
Santa Cruz organic juices
Mountain Sun organic juices
Fruit

Sweet Treats
New Morning Graham Crackers: Honey, Chocolate, Cinnamon

Reasons to Buy Organically

1. Because children are smaller and need high-energy food for growth, they receive four times the exposure to pesticides as an adult. Eating organically will affect their health in the future.

2. Organic farmers pay attention to the soil they grow their produce in. Conventional farmers use chemical fertilizers, ignoring the soil ecosystem, which is eroding much faster than it is built up naturally.

3. Pesticides used in conventional farming are contaminating the water, killing sea life and other important organisms.

4. Organic produce travels a shorter distance from the farm to your plate, so fruits and vegetables can be picked riper, containing more vitamins.

5. Pesticides have been linked to cancer, birth defects, nerve damage, and genetic mutations.

6. A Cancer Institute study found that farmers exposed to herbicides have a six times greater risk than nonfarmers of contracting cancer.

7. Organic foods aren't really more expensive in the end. Conventional food prices fool you into thinking they are cheaper, but have hidden costs such as pesticide regulation and testing, hazardous waste disposal and cleanup, damage to the environment, and medical costs.

8. Conventional farms plant large areas of land with the same crop every year. This robs the soil of minerals and nutrients. To replace the minerals, farmers use chemical fertilizers in large amounts, which kills wildlife and soil organisms.

9. Organic produce just tastes better.

Appendix

Vitamin A

FRUITS	% VITAMIN A
Apricot	45
Cantaloupe	100
Dried Apricots	50
Mango	40
Watermelon	20

VEGETABLES	% VITAMIN A
Carrot	70
Collards	50
Hot Chili Peppers	80
Leaf Lettuce	50
Mustard Greens	90
Romaine Lettuce	20
Spinach	70
Sweet Potato	40
Tomato	20

Vitamin C

FRUITS	% VITAMIN C
Apricot	20
Blackberries	50
Cantaloupe	80
Carambola	30
Gooseberries	60
Grapefruit	110
Grapes	25
Honeydew Melon	45
Kiwifruit	240
Lemon	40
Lime	35
Orange	130
Papaya	150
Pineapple	25
Plum	20
Prickly Pear	25
Pomelo	130
Raspberries	40
Strawberries	160
Tangerine	50
Watermelon	25

VEGETABLES	% VITAMIN C
Bell Pepper	190
Broccoli	220
Brussels Sprouts	120
Cabbage (Green)	70
Cauliflower	100
Collards	30
Green Cauliflower	90
Hot Chili Peppers	170
Mustard Greens	100
Okra	20
Onions	20
Potato	45
Radishes	30
Red Cabbage	70
Rutabagas	90
Spinach	25
Summer Squash	30
Sweet Potato	30
Tomato	40
Yellow Snap Beans	20

Calcium in Foods

Vegetables:	Calcium (mg)
Broccoli (1 cup, boiled)	178
Brussels sprouts (8 sprouts)	56
Carrots (2 medium)	38
Cauliflower (1 cup, boiled)	34
Celery (1 cup, boiled)	54
Collards (1 cup, boiled)	148
Kale (1 cup, boiled)	94
Onions (1 cup, boiled)	58
Potato, baked (1 medium)	20
Romaine lettuce (1 cup)	20
Squash, butternut (1 cup, boiled)	84
Sweet potato (1 cup, boiled)	70

Legumes:

Chickpeas	78
Great Northern beans (1 cup, boiled)	121
Green beans (1 cup, boiled)	58
Kidney beans (1 cup, boiled)	50
Lentils (1 cup, boiled)	37
Lima beans (1 cup, boiled)	52
Navy beans (1 cup, boiled)	128
Peas, green (1 cup, boiled)	44
Pinto beans (1 cup, boiled)	82
Soybeans (1 cup, boiled)	175
Turtle beans, black (1 cup, boiled)	103
Tofu (½ cup)	258
Vegetarian baked beans (1 cup)	128
Wax beans (1 cup, canned)	174
White beans (1 cup, boiled)	161

Grains:	Calcium (mg)
Brown rice (cooked, 1 cup)	23
Corn bread (one 2-ounce piece)	133
Corn tortilla (1 medium)	42
English muffin (1 medium)	92
Pancake mix (¼ cup, 3 pancakes)	140
Pita bread (1 piece)	31
Wheat bread (1 slice)	30
Wheat flour, all-purpose (1 cup)	22
Wheat flour, calcium enriched (1 cup)	238
Whole wheat flour (1 cup)	49

Fruits:

Apple (1 medium)	10
Banana (1 medium)	7
Figs, dried (10 medium)	269
Orange, navel (1 medium)	56
Orange juice, calcium-fortified (1 cup)	300
Organic orange juice (Horizon)	300
Pear (1 medium)	19
Raisins (⅔ cup)	53

Other Calcium-Rich Foods:

Blackstrap molasses (2 tablespoons)	274
Rice Dream (8 ounces)	300
Sesame seeds (½ cup)	702
Silk cultured soy yogurt (6 ounces)	500
Silk soy milk (8 ounces)	300
Soy cheese slices (1 slice)	200

Items That Affect Your Child's Brain

Foods	Dairy products, dairy components (casein, lactalbumin, whey, lactose), chocolate, egg whites, wheat, corn, oranges, and peanuts.
Sweeteners	Sugar (cane or beet) and refined starches (corn syrup, cornstarch, modified food starch, maltodextrin), high-fructose corn syrup, all artificial sweeteners (NutraSweet, Equal, Sweet'n Low, Sucralose, Acesulfame-K).
Additives	All artificial colors, but especially red dye #3 (erythrosine) and yellow dye #5 (tartrazine), which are the most studied and proven to exacerbate ADHD.
Flavors	MSG, vanillin, and smoke flavoring are the most common; salt, sodium-containing agents, and sodium or potassium phosphate (buffering agents).
Preservatives	BHA, BHT, TBHQ, sodium benzoate, calcium propionate, nitrates, nitrites, sulfites, and citric acid.
Beverages	All caffeinated tea, coffee, and sodas; sweetened fruit juices and beverages and all others that contain phosphates.
Fats	All hydrogenated and partially hydrogenated fats, mono- and diglycerides, Olestra, Olean, tropical fats (palm, palm kernel, coconut), cottonseed oil.

Source: Zimmerman, *The A.D.D. Nutrition Solution*

Major Risks to Children

Cases of accidental ingestion in young children were reported by the American Association of Poison Control Centers as follows for 1998:

Cosmetics and personal care products.	157,551
Cleaning substances	129,441
Analgesics	89,985
Plants	84,185
Foreign bodies	73,983
Cough and cold preparations	64,761
Topicals	63,623
Insecticides, pesticides, rodenticides	46,447
Vitamins	39,396
Antimicrobials	36,597
Gastrointestinal preparations	35,391
Arts/crafts/office supplies	29,898
Hydrocarbons	26,018
Antihistamines	22,854
Hormones and hormone antagonists	22,655

Source: *Good Medicine,* vol. 9, No. 1, Winter 2000

Educational Problems in Children

1. A child must be able to perceive the stimuli presented, determine what's demanded, and then concentrate her attention on a specific problem or stimulus.

2. She must be able to organize incoming information in relation to past knowledge and then code it for future retrieval (memory).

3. A child must have some ability to communicate with others (language, verbal and written).

4. She must be motivated to perform (without performance, there can be no indication that learning has taken place).

5. A child must display conduct appropriate to a given situation. That is, she must behave properly with teachers and classmates.

Tips for Parents on Children's Allergies

All children with allergies are not the same.

Some children may be allergic to a food item, while others are allergic to something else entirely. There are various degrees to which each child will be allergic as well. If your child has allergies, make sure his teacher and school nurse have a list of all possible foods that can cause him to have a reaction.

Watch out for hidden ingredients or foods with different names.

Always read the ingredients on food packaging. Many times you will not know that a product contains trace amounts of an ingredient that your child is allergic to. Also, be aware that if your child is allergic to a food like sugar, he will not be able to have corn syrup, dextrose, glucose, fructose, or honey. The names of many foods have synonyms.

Never force a child to taste food.

If your child tells you that he does not feel well if he eats a particular food, listen to him.

Plan ahead.

Ask your child's teacher to make you aware if the class will be celebrating any birthdays or holidays so that you can make alternate food arrangements if they are needed. Or volunteer to be the class parent or help prepare for celebrations in your child's class so that ingredients can be monitored.

Reward creatively.

Food isn't the only way to reward your child for a job well done. Stickers, books, or a trip to the arcade will be just as effective.

Don't pity the allergic child.

Your child knows how he feels when he eats something that he is allergic to. He will usually do the right thing. His allergies actually help in making decisions and building character. Admire children for their strength.

Ethyl Methyl Key

A—probably carcinogenic (cancer causing)
B—caused serious side effects in lab animals
C—may contribute to heart or lung disease
D—may contribute to gastrointestinal, liver, or kidney disease
E—may cause birth defects
F—associated with nausea or vomiting
G—toxic
H—adversely affects the central nervous system
I—may adversely affect brain function and memory
J—may weaken the immune system
K—causes common allergic reactions (runny nose, rash, etc.)
L—not sufficiently tested
M—relatively minor side effects
N—serious side effects from abnormally large doses
P—allergic reactions for some
GRAS—generally regarded as safe by the FDA. (This doesn't necessarily mean it's safe. For example, cyclamates were once on this list. And believe it or not, BHA, BHT, and MSG are *still* on it.)

Category One (Most Dangerous)

Acesulfame-K: (A, B)
Acesulfame-potassium: (A, B)
Acetal: (C)
Acetaldehyde: (H) GRAS
Alkyl gallate: (D)
Allyl sulfide: (C, D)
Aloe extract: (D)
Aluminum: (D, I, L)
Ammonium: (D)
Amyl acetate: (H)
Amyl alcohol: (G)
Animal or vegetable shortening: (C)
Artemisia: (D, H)
Artificial color FD&C: (A, H, I)
Aspartame: (E, H, I)
Aspergillus oryzae: (A)
Azo dyes: (C, D)

Benzyl alcohol: (F)
BHA: (A, B, D, E, J) GRAS
BHT: (A, B, D, E, J) GRAS
Biphenyl: (F)
Blue No. 1: (A, C, K, L)
Blue No. 2: (B, C, K)
Boric acid: (G)
Borneol: (D, H)
Brominated vegetable oil: (C, D, E)
Butylated hydroxyanisole-BHA: (A, B, D, E, J) GRAS
Butylated hydroxytoluene-BHT: (A, B, D, E, J) GRAS
Caffeine: addictive drug (C, D, E, H, I) GRAS
Calcium chloride: (C, D) GRAS
Calcium glucanate: (C, D) GRAS

Calcium lactate: (C, D) GRAS
Camphor oil: (E)
Carboxymethylcellulose: (B) GRAS
Carvacrol: (C, G)
Chlorine dioxide: (A)
Cinnamaldehyde: (D, K) GRAS
Coal tar dyes: (C, D, K)
Cocoa: contains caffeine
Corn sugar: (C, D, H, M) GRAS
Corn syrup: (C, D, H, M)
Cyclamates: (A)
Dimethylpolysiloxane: (D)
Dioctyl sodium sulfosuccinate (DDS): (D, E, L)
Diphenyl: (F, K)
Disodium phosphate: (C, D) GRAS
Ethyl vanillin: (B) GRAS
FD&C Blue No. 1: (A, C, K, L)
FD&C Blue No. 2: (B, C, K)
FD&C Citrus Red No. 2: (A)
FD&C Green No. 3: (A)
FD&C Red No. 3: (B)
FD&C Red No. 40: (H)
FD&C Yellow No. 5: (D, K)
FD&C Yellow No. 6: (A, B)
Formaldehyde: (A, E, G)
Free glutamates: (I)
Fructose: (C, D)
Glycerin: (F) GRAS
Heptylparaben: (E, L)
High fructose corn syrup: (C, D) GRAS
Hydrogenated vegetable oil: (A, C)
Hydrogen peroxide: (A) GRAS
Hydrolyzed vegetable protein: (H, I)
Imitation flavoring: (D, H)

Isolated soy protein: (F, I) if it contains nitrites
Leavening: may contain BHA & BHT
Mannitol: (D, F, L)
MSG-Monosodium glutamate: (E, D, H, I, K)
Nitrates: (A) Very dangerous carcinogen!
Nitrates: (A, F, I) Also very dangerous!
Olean and Olestra: (D)
Partially hydrogenated vegetable oil: (A, C)
Phenylglycidate: (B)
Phenylmethyl cyclosiloxane: (B, D)
Phosphates: (D)
Polyxyethylene stearate: (D, K)
Potassium acetate: (D)
Potassium alginate: (C, D)
Potassium benzoate: (C, D, K) GRAS
Potassium bisulfite: (C, D)
Potassium bromate: (A, D, H)
Potassium chloride: (C, D, F) GRAS
Potassium nitrate: (A)—aka nitrates
Potassium nitrite: (A, F, I)—aka nitrites
Quinine: (E, L)
Saccharin: (A) Very dangerous!
Salatrim: (F, L)
Sodium acetate: (C, D)
Sodium alginate: (C, D, E)
Sodium aluminum sulfate: (B, I)
Sodium bisulfite: (C, G)
Sodium carbonate: (C, D)
Sodium nitrate: (A)—aka nitrates
Sodium nitrite: (A, F, I)—aka nitrites
Sodium polyphosphate: (D)
Vegetable shortening: (A, C)
Whey: dairy product: (C, D)
Whey protein concentrate: dairy product: (C, D)

Category Two

Unclear (as in untested) or associated with less serious problems.

Acacia gum: (K, L) GRAS
Acetate: (N)
Acetic acid: (M) GRAS
Agar-agar: (N) GRAS
Alpha tocopherol acetate: (N)
Amylases: (P)
Angelica: (M) GRAS
Arabinogalactan: (L)
Ascorbic acid: (M) GRAS
Ascorbyl palmitate: (M) GRAS
Baking powder: (may contain aluminum)
Barley malt: (M, P)
Benzaldehyde: (H, J, M)
Benzoate of soda: (D, K) GRAS
Benzoic acid: (D, K) GRAS
Benzyl acetate: (D)
Benzyl formate: (N)
Bergamot: (M)
Blackstrap molasses: (M)
Brown algae: (L) GRAS
Calcium phosphate: (D) GRAS
Calcium sulfate: (B) GRAS
Capsicum: (D) GRAS
Carmine: (L)
Carob bean gum: (L, P) GRAS
Casein: (P) GRAS
Castor oil: (N)
Citric acid: (M) GRAS
Clove bud oil: (M)
Clove leaf oil: (M)
Clover: (M)
Coconut oil: (C)
Corn gluten: (P) GRAS
Cornstarch: (K, M) GRAS
Dill: (M) GRAS
Dill oil: (N)
Disodium guanylate: (L, M, P)
Disodium inosinate: (L, M, P)
Erythorbic acid: (K, P) GRAS

Ethyl alcohol: (C, N)–fatal in large doses GRAS
Formic acid: (M)
Fruit juice concentrate: (D, P)
Fumaric acid: (K, L, P) GRAS
Glucose: (M)
Gluten: (K, P)
Invert sugar: (M, P) GRAS
L-ascorbic acid: (D, N)
Licorice: (C, N) GRAS
Mace/nutmeg: (N) Very dangerous hallucinogenic drug in high doses GRAS
Magnesium compounds: (P) GRAS
Menadione: (M)
Modified food starch: (L) GRAS
Mono- and diglycerides: (C, D, K, L) GRAS
Niacin: (M) GRAS
Nickel: (M, N) GRAS
Nitrous oxide: (B, M, P) GRAS
Paprika: (N) GRAS
Parabens: (L) GRAS
Pectins: (M) GRAS
Saffron: (N) GRAS
St. John's bread gum: (K, L) GRAS
Salicylates: (P)
Salt: (C, D, P) GRAS
Silica: (D)
Sodium acetate: (C, D) GRAS
Sodium alginate: (C, D) GRAS
Sodium chloride: (C, D, P) GRAS
Sodium sulfate: (C, D)
Stearic acid: may come from hydrogenated oils GRAS
Sucrose: (D, M) GRAS
Turmeric: (M) GRAS
Vegetable gum: (L)
Vitamin A: (N) GRAS
Vitamin A acetate: (N) GRAS
Vitamin A palmitate: (N) GRAS

Vitamin D$_2$: (N) GRAS
Vitamin D$_3$: (N) GRAS
Wheat gluten: (P) GRAS

Xanthan gum: (D, M)
Zinc chloride: (K, M) GRAS
Zinc sulfate: (B, D) GRAS

Category Three

(Currently considered safe and/or nutritional.)

Acetoin GRAS
Acetyl methylcarbinol GRAS
Aconitic acid GRAS
Adiptic acid GRAS
Alfalfa GRAS
Allspice GRAS
Annatto
Baker's yeast glycan
Baker's yeast protein
Beta-carotene GRAS
Biotin GRAS
Calcium glycerophosphate GRAS
Calcium pyrophosphate GRAS
Carbon dioxide GRAS
Carotene GRAS
Choline bitartrate GRAS

Choline chloride GRAS
Decanal GRAS
Dillseed
Ergocalciferol
Ethyl butyrate GRAS
Ethyl heptanoate GRAS
Folcin
Folic acid
Fruit pectin
Garlic GRAS
Ground limestone GRAS
Inositol GRAS
L-cysteine GRAS
L-lysine
Lactoflavin

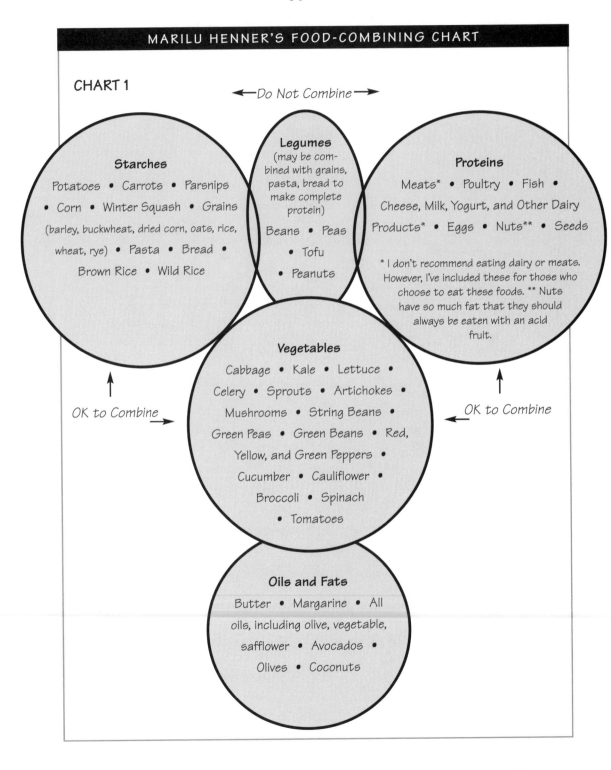

MARILU HENNER'S FOOD-COMBINING CHART

CHART 1

←— Do Not Combine —→

Starches

Potatoes • Carrots • Parsnips • Corn • Winter Squash • Grains (barley, buckwheat, dried corn, oats, rice, wheat, rye) • Pasta • Bread • Brown Rice • Wild Rice

Legumes
(may be combined with grains, pasta, bread to make complete protein)

Beans • Peas • Tofu • Peanuts

Proteins

Meats* • Poultry • Fish • Cheese, Milk, Yogurt, and Other Dairy Products* • Eggs • Nuts** • Seeds

* I don't recommend eating dairy or meats. However, I've included these for those who choose to eat these foods. ** Nuts have so much fat that they should always be eaten with an acid fruit.

↑

OK to Combine →

Vegetables

Cabbage • Kale • Lettuce • Celery • Sprouts • Artichokes • Mushrooms • String Beans • Green Peas • Green Beans • Red, Yellow, and Green Peppers • Cucumber • Cauliflower • Broccoli • Spinach • Tomatoes

↑

← OK to Combine

Oils and Fats

Butter • Margarine • All oils, including olive, vegetable, safflower • Avocados • Olives • Coconuts

DO NOT COMBINE FOODS FROM CHART 1 AND 2

CHART 2

← OK to Combine →

Acid Fruits

Grapefruits • Oranges • Lemons • Limes • Strawberries • Cranberries • Kiwis • Pineapples

Sub-Acid Fruits

Apples • Apricots • Blackberries • Cherries • Peaches • Plums • Pears • Raspberries • Mangoes • Nectarines • Grapes • Papayas

Sweet Fruits

Bananas • Plantains • Dates • Persimmons • Figs • Prunes • Raisins • Dried Fruits

Do not combine with other foods

Melons

Cantaloupe • Honeydew • Watermelon • Casaba • Christmas • Crenshaw

Do not combine with other foods

113 Ways Sugar Can Ruin Your Health

In addition to throwing off the body's homeostasis, excess sugar may have a number of other significant consequences. The following listing of some of sugar's negative metabolic effects was culled from a variety of medical journals and other scientific publications.

1. Sugar can suppress the immune system.
2. Sugar can upset the body's mineral balance.
3. Sugar can cause hyperactivity, anxiety, concentration difficulties, and crankiness in children.
4. Sugar can cause drowsiness and decreased activity in children.
5. Sugar can adversely affect children's school grades.
6. Sugar can produce a significant rise in triglycerides.
7. Sugar contributes to a weakened defense against bacterial infection.
8. Sugar can cause kidney damage.
9. Sugar can reduce helpful high-density cholesterol (HDLs).
10. Sugar can promote an elevation of harmful cholesterol (LDLs).
11. Sugar may lead to chromium deficiency.
12. Sugar can cause copper deficiency.
13. Sugar interferes with absorption of calcium and magnesium.
14. Sugar may lead to cancer of the breast, ovaries, prostate, and rectum.
15. Sugar can cause colon cancer, with an increased risk in women.
16. Sugar can be a risk factor in gallbladder cancer.
17. Sugar can increase fasting levels of blood glucose.
18. Sugar can weaken eyesight.
19. Sugar raises the level of a neurotransmitter called serotonin, which can narrow blood vessels.
20. Sugar can cause hypoglycemia.
21. Sugar can produce an acidic stomach.
22. Sugar can raise adrenaline levels in children.
23. Sugar can increase the risk of coronary heart disease.
24. Sugar can speed the aging process, causing wrinkles and gray hair.
25. Sugar can lead to alcoholism.
26. Sugar can promote tooth decay.
27. Sugar can contribute to weight gain and obesity.
28. High intake of sugar increases the risk of Crohn's disease and ulcerative colitis.
29. Sugar can cause a raw, inflamed intestinal tract in persons with gastric or duodenal ulcers.
30. Sugar can cause arthritis.
31. Sugar can cause asthma.
32. Sugar can cause candidiasis (yeast infection).
33. Sugar can lead to the formation of gallstones.
34. Sugar can lead to the formation of kidney stones.
35. Sugar can cause ischemic heart disease.
36. Sugar can cause appendicitis.

37. Sugar can exacerbate the symptoms of multiple sclerosis.
38. Sugar can indirectly cause hemorrhoids.
39. Sugar can cause varicose veins.
40. Sugar can elevate glucose and insulin responses in oral contraception users.
41. Sugar can lead to periodontal disease.
42. Sugar can contribute to osteoporosis.
43. Sugar contributes to saliva acidity.
44. Sugar can cause a decrease in insulin sensitivity.
45. Sugar leads to decreased glucose tolerance.
46. Sugar can decrease growth hormone.
47. Sugar can increase total cholesterol.
48. Sugar can increase systolic blood pressure.
49. Sugar can change the structure of protein, causing interference with protein absorption.
50. Sugar causes food allergies.
51. Sugar can contribute to diabetes.
52. Sugar can cause toxemia during pregnancy.
53. Sugar can contribute to eczema in children.
54. Sugar can cause cardiovascular disease.
55. Sugar can impair the structure of DNA.
56. Sugar can cause cataracts.
57. Sugar can cause emphysema.
58. Sugar can cause atherosclerosis.
59. Sugar can cause free radical formation in the bloodstream.
60. Sugar lowers the enzymes' ability to function.
61. Sugar can cause loss of tissue elasticity and function.
62. Sugar can cause liver cells to divide, increasing the size of the liver.
63. Sugar can increase the amount of fat in the liver.
64. Sugar can increase kidney size and produce pathological changes in the kidney.
65. Sugar can overstress the pancreas, causing damage.
66. Sugar can increase the body's fluid retention.
67. Sugar can cause constipation.
68. Sugar can cause myopia (nearsightedness).
69. Sugar can compromise the lining of the capillaries.
70. Sugar can cause hypertension.
71. Sugar can cause headaches, including migraines.
72. Sugar can cause an increase in delta, alpha, and theta brain waves, which can alter the mind's ability to think clearly.
73. Sugar can cause depression.
74. Sugar can increase insulin responses in those consuming high sugar diets compared to low sugar diets.
75. Sugar increases bacterial fermentation in the colon.
76. Sugar can cause hormonal imbalance.
77. Sugar can increase blood platelet adhesiveness, which increases the risk of blood clots.
78. Sugar can increase the risk of Alzheimer's disease.
79. Sugar can cause an increase in delta, alpha, and theta brain waves.

80. Sugar can cause depression.
81. Sugar increases risk of gastric cancer.
82. Sugar causes dyspepsia (indigestion).
83. Sugar can increase your risk of getting gout.
84. The ingestion of sugar can increase the levels of glucose in an oral glucose tolerance test over the ingestion of complex carbohydrates.
85. Sugar can increase the insulin responses in humans consuming high sugar diets compared to low sugar diets.
86. Sugar increases bacterial fermentation in the colon.
87. Sugar increases the risk of colon cancer in women.
88. There is a greater risk for Crohn's Disease with people who have a high intake of sugar.
89. Sugar can cause platelet adhesiveness.
90. Sugar can cause hormonal imbalance.
91. Sugar can lead to the formation of kidney stones.
92. Sugar can lead the hypothalamus to become highly sensitive to a large variety of stimuli.
93. Sugar can lead to dizziness.
94. High sucrose diets significantly increase serum insulin.
95. High sucrose diets of subjects with peripheral vascular disease significantly increase platelet adhesion.
96. High sugar diets can lead to biliary tract cancer.
97. High sugar diets tend to be lower in antioxidant micro nutrients.
98. High sugar consumption by pregnant adolescents is associated with a twofold increase risk for delivering a small-for-gestational age (SGA) infant.
99. High sugar consumption can lead to substantial decrease in gestation duration among adolescents with high sugar diets.
100. Sugar slows food's travel time through the gastrointestinal tract.
101. Sugar increases the concentration of bile acids in stools, and bacterial enzymes in the colon can modify bile to produce cancer-causing compounds and colon cancer.
102. Sugar is associated with a substantial decrease in normal time of gestation among adolescents.
103. Sugar can cause a depletion of chromium which is tied to the development and progression of nearsightedness.
104. Sugar can be a risk factor of gallbladder disease.
105. Sugar is an addictive substance.
106. Sugar can be intoxicating, similar to alcohol.
107. Sugar can exacerbate PMS.
108. Sugar suppresses lymphocytes.
109. Decrease in sugar can increase emotional stability.
110. The body changes sugar two to five times more fat in the bloodstream than it does starch.
111. Sugar can cause inappropriate behavior and decreased performance in children.
112. Sugar can worsen the symptoms of children with attention deficit disorder (ADD).
113. The sugar in chewing gum can cause dental cavities.

Nancy Appleton, author of *Lick the Sugar Habit*

Bibliography

Alexander, D., and L. Goldman. *Investing in Our Future: A National Research Initiative for Children for the 21st Century.* Washington, DC: Office of Science and Technology Policy, 1997.

Anderson, Nina, and Howard Peiper. *A.D.D. The Natural Approach: Help for Children with Attention Deficit Disorder and Hyperactivity.* East Canaan, CT: Safe Goods, 1996.

Bailar, J.L., and H.L. Gornik. "Cancer Undefeated." *New England Journal of Medicine,* 336:1569–1574 (1997).

Baird, D.B., and A.J. Wilcox. "Cigarette Smoking Associated with Delayed Conception." *JAMA,* 253:2979–2983 (1985).

Bearer, G.F. "How Are Children Different from Adults?" *Environmental Health Perspective* 103 (Supplement 6):7–12 (1995).

Bellinger D., A. Leviton, C. Waternaux, and H.L. Needleman. "Longitudinal Analyses of Prenatal and Postnatal Exposure and Early Cognitive Development." *New England Journal of Medicine* 315:1037–1043 (1987).

Bethel, May. *The Healing Power of Natural Foods.* North Hollywood, CA: Wilshire Book Co., 1978.

Block, Dr. Mary Ann. *No More Ritalin: Treating ADHD Without Drugs.* Boston: Houghton Mifflin, 2001.

Brinkley, Ginny, Linda Goldberg, and Janice Kukar. *Your Child's First Journey: A Guide to Prepared Birth from Pregnancy to Parenthood.* Garden City Park, NY: Avery Publishing Group, Inc., 1988.

Brody, Jane E. *The New York Times Book of Health: How to Feel Fitter, Eat Better and Live Longer.* New York: Random House, 1997.

Caplan, Frank. *The First Twelve Months of Life: Your Baby's Growth Month by Month.* New York: Grosset & Dunlap, 1971.

Bibliography

Clinton, Ellyn. *Child of Mine: Feeding with Love and Good Sense Protection of Children from Environmental Health Risks and Safety Risks*. Washington, DC: U.S. GPO. Executive Order #13045, April 21, 1997.

Colborn T., D. Dumanoski, and J.P. Myers. *Our Stolen Future*. New York: Dutton, 1996.

Cowley, Geoffrey. "Cannibals to Cows: The Path of a Deadly Disease:" *Newsweek* (March 12, 2001): 53–61.

DesMaisons, Kathleen, Ph.D. *Addictive Nutrition: Potatoes Not Prozac*. New York: Simon & Schuster, 1999.

Duncan, Alice Likowski, D.C. *Your Healthy Child: A Guide to Natural Health Care for Children*. Los Angeles: Jeremy P. Tarcher, Inc., 1991.

Economist. "The Power of Suggestion," May 18, 1996, pp. S4–S5.

Eisenberg, Arlene, Heidi Eisenberg Murkoff, and Sandee Eisenberg Hathaway, R.N., B.S.N., *What to Expect When You're Expecting*. New York: Workman Publishing, 1984.

Feingold, Ben F., M.D. *Why Your Child Is Hyperactive*. New York: Random House, 1975.

Garland, Anne Witte, with Mothers and Others for a Livable Planet. *The Way We Grow: Good-Sense Solutions for Protecting Our Families from Pesticides in Food*. New York: Berkley Books, 1993.

Gordon, Jay, M.D., with Antonia Barnes Boyle. *Good Food Today, Great Kids Tomorrow: 50 Things You Can Do for Healthy, Happy Children*. Studio City, CA: Michael Wiese Productions, 1994.

Green, Martin I. *A Sigh of Relief: The First-Aid Handbook for Childhood Emergencies*. New York: Bantam Books, 1977.

Haughton, Emma. *Drinking, Smoking, and Other Drugs*. Austin, TX: Raintree Steck-Vaughn Publishers, 2000.

Hausman, Patricia, and Judith Benn Hurley. *The Healing Foods*. Emmaus, PA: Rodale Press, 1989.

Jacobson, Michael F., Ph.D., and Sarah Fritschner. *Fast-food Guide*. New York: Workman Publishing, 1991.

Jensen, Bernard. *Creating a Magic Kitchen*. Provo, UT: BiWorld Publishers, Inc., 1973.

Jones, Anita, M.P.H., Esther Hill, Ph.D., and Erica Bohm, M.S. *Healthy Dining in Los Angeles*. San Diego, CA: Healthy Dining Publications—Accents on Health, Inc., 1998.

Katherine, Anne, M.A. *Anatomy of a Food Addiction: The Brain Chemistry of Overeating*. Carlsbad, CA: Gurze Books, 1991.

Kitzinger, Sheila. *Breastfeeding Your Baby*. New York: Dorling Kindersley, 1989.

Klapper, Michael, M.D. *Pregnancy, Children, and the Vegan Diet*. Maui, HI:1987.

Klavan, Ellen. *The Vegetarian Factfinder*. New York: The Little Bookroom, 1996.

Kushi, Michio, and Aveline Kushi, with Edward Esko and Wendy Esko. *Raising Healthy Kids*. Garden City Park, NY: Avery Publishing Group, 1994.

Landrigan, Philip J., and Joy Carlson. "Environmental Policy and Children's Health," in *The Future of Children*, Vol. 5. No. 2, Summer/Fall 1995.

Leff, Mechal "No More Meat?" *Consumer Reports on Health* (October 1995): 109–112.

McNeal, James U. *Kids as Customers: A Handbook of Marketing to Children*. New York: Lexington Books, 1992.

Miller, Saul, with Jo Anne Miller. *Food for Thought: A New Look at Food and Behavior.* Englewood Cliffs, NJ: Prentice-Hall, Inc., 1979.

Muramoto, Naboru. *Healing Ourselves.* New York: Avon, 1973.

Null, Gary. *The Complete Guide to Health and Nutrition: A Sourcebook for a Healthier Life.* New York: Random House, Inc., 2000.

Page, Linda Rector, N.D., Ph.D. *Healthy Healing: A Guide to Self-Healing for Everyone.* Carmel Valley, CA: Healthy Healing Publications, 1998.

Rapp, Doris J., M.D. *Is This Your Child's World?* New York: Bantam Books, 1996.

Ridgway, Roy. *Asthma: The Natural Way.* Shaftesbury, Dorset, England. Element, 1994.

Sahley, Billie Jay, Ph.D., C.N.C. *Control Hyperactivity A.D.D. Naturally.* San Antonio, TX: Pain and Stress Publications, 2000.

Samuels, Mike, M.D., and Nancy Samuels. *The Well Baby Book.* New York: Summit Books, 1991.

Schaefer, Valorie Lee. *The Care and Keeping of You: The Body Book for Girls.* Middleton, WI: Pleasant Company Publications, 1998.

Schlosser, Eric. *Fast Food Nation: The Dark Side of the All-American Meal.* Boston, MA: Houghton Mifflin Company, 2001.

Scott, Julian, Ph.D. *Natural Medicine for Children: Drug-Free Health Care for Children from Birth to Age Twelve.* New York: Avon Books, 1990.

Simontacchi, Carol. *The Crazy Makers: How the Food Industry Is Destroying Our Brains and Harming Our Children.* New York: Jeremy P. Tarcher, 2000.

Tenney, Deanne. *Children's Herbal Health.* Pleasant Grove, UT: Woodland Publishing, 1996.

Tenney, Louise. *Today's Herbal Health for Children: A Comprehensive Guide to Understanding Nutrition and Herbal Medicine for Children.* Grove, UT: Woodland Publishing, Inc.

Ullman, Dana, M.P.H. *Homeopathic Medicine for Children and Infants.* New York: Jeremy P. Tarcher, 1992.

Weiner, Ellen. *Taking Food Allergies to School.* Valley Park, MO: JayJo Books, 1999.

Weiss, Rick. "What's the Matter with Milk?" *Health* (January/February 1993): 18–20.

Whitaker, Julian M., M.D. *Reversing Diabetes.* New York: Warner Books, 1987.

Zand, Janet, OMD, L.AC. and Rachel Walton, R.N., and Bob Rountree, M.D. *Smart Medicine for a Healthier Child: A Practical A-to-Z Reference to Natural and Conventional Treatments for Infants and Children.* Garden City Park, NY: Avery Publishing Group, 1994.

Zimmerman, Marcia, C.N. *The A.D.D. Nutrition Solution: A Drug-Free 30-Day Plan.* New York: Henry Holt & Co., 1999.

ReganBooks *An Imprint of HarperCollinsPublishers*

Books by Marilu Henner:

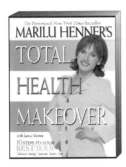

MARILU HENNER'S TOTAL HEALTH MAKEOVER

ISBN 0-06-098878-9 (paperback); ISBN 0-06-109828-0 (mass market); ISBN 0-694-51927-8 (audio)

With irrepressible enthusiasm and humor, Marilu presents practical advice on diet myths, toxic foods, mood swings, food combining, and her unique, flexible, down-to-earth 10-step life plan. With *Marilu Henner's Total Health Makeover* you can free yourself from diets and disease-causing toxins, boost your energy, lower and maintain your weight, and change your outlook in as little as three weeks.

THE 30 DAY TOTAL HEALTH MAKEOVER

Everything You Need to Do to Change Your Body,
Your Health, and Your Life in 30 Amazing Days

ISBN 0-06-103133-X (paperback)

This inspirational how-to guide for total health living and your B.E.S.T. body in just 30 days includes day-to-day goals; strategies for success; recipes for breakfast, lunch, and dinner; shopping lists; exercise ideas; and what to feed the kids.

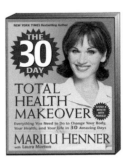

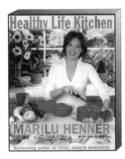

HEALTHY LIFE KITCHEN

ISBN 0-06-098857-6 (paperback)

Marilu Henner provides a delicious collection of healthy recipes that will help readers change their bodies and their lives forever. Created by Marilu and her favorite chefs from restaurants all over the world, these delectable breakfasts, lunches, dinners, desserts, and snacks will raise healthy cuisine to a new level of taste and ease. There is even a "healthy junkfood" section for converting naughty treats into nutritious recipes.

I REFUSE TO RAISE A BRAT

ISBN 0-06-098730-8 (paperback); ISBN 0-694-52129-9 (audio)

Supermom Marilu Henner and renowned psychoanalyst Dr. Ruth Sharon provide simple and straightforward advice on how to raise secure, happy, and self-reliant children. *I Refuse to Raise a Brat* teaches readers how to distinguish between overgratification and love, break the pattern of overindulgence, and offer children the balance of frustration and gratification they need.

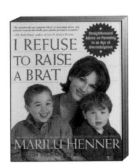

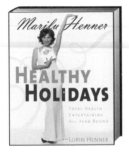

HEALTHY HOLIDAYS

Total Health Entertaining All Year Round

ISBN 0-06-039363-7 (hardcover)

Maintaining a healthy lifestyle throughout the year is tough enough, but when special occasions roll around, most people throw up their hands and dig in with abandon—knowing that they'll regret it later. Marilu Henner offers another choice. In her new book, *Healthy Holidays*, Marilu shows us how easy and fun it is to prepare healthy meals for you and your family on special occasions and holidays year-round.

Want to receive notice of author events and new books by Marilu Henner?
Sign up for Marilu Henner's AuthorTracker at www.AuthorTracker.com